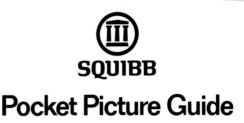

SQUIBB

Pocket Picture Guide

CARDIOLOGY

Adam D. Timmis
MD, MRCP

Senior Registrar,
Department of Cardiology,
Guy's Hospital,
London, UK

**Presented as a service to medicine by
E.R. Squibb and Sons Limited**

Produced and Published by
Gower Medical Publishing · London · New York · 1985

Acknowledgements

The author would like to thank the following colleagues for providing illustrative material: Dr. L. Adams, Guy's Hospital, London (Figs. 194, 197); Prof. A. E. Becker, Department of Pathology, University of Amsterdam, Amsterdam (Fig. 42); Dr. D. A. Chamberlain, Royal Sussex County Hospital, Brighton (Fig. 152); Dr. J. C. P. Crick, Guy's Hospital, London (Figs. 143, 151, 184); Dr. C. E. Essed, Department of Pathology, Erasmus University, Rotterdam (Fig. 101); M. Monaghan, King's College Hospital, London (Figs. 41, 73, 88, 99, 124, 211); Dr. S. Rankin, Guy's Hospital, London (Figs. 10, 201); Dr. J. Reidy, Guy's Hospital, London (Figs. 17, 193, 206); Dr. B. Timmis, Whittington Hospital, London (Figs. 19, 128, 196, 205).

ISBN 0-906923-45-X

Project Editor: Fiona Carr
Design: Helen Udesen
Cover: Max Dyson
Illustration: Pamela Corfield

Printed in Italy by Imago Publishing Ltd.

Contents

The Normal Heart

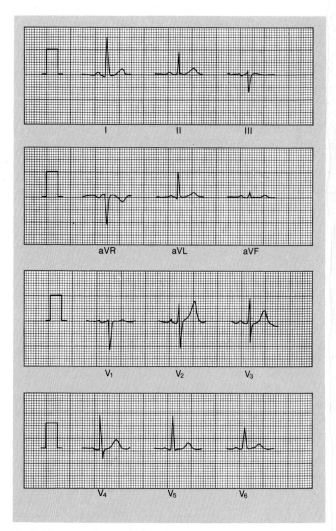

Fig.1 Electrocardiogram (ECG). This is a record of the electrical activity of the heart recorded at the skin surface. Six *bipolar* leads (I to aVF) and six *unipolar* leads (V1 to V6) are usually displayed. The paper speed is 25mm per second such that each small square (1mm) represents 0.04 seconds and each large square (5mm) represents 0.20 seconds. The square wave is a calibration signal: 1cm vertical deflection = 1mV. A calibration signal should be included with every 12 lead ECG recording.

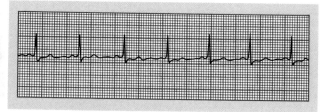

Fig.2 Sinus rhythm (lead II). The sinus node is the pacemaker of the normal heart. It depolarises spontaneously at regular intervals which determine the heart rate. The sinus node is influenced by a variety of neurohumoral factors, particularly vagal and sympathetic activity which respectively slow and quicken the heart rate. Each sinus discharge produces atrial depolarisation (P wave) followed by ventricular depolarisation (QRS complex) and ventricular repolarisation (T wave). This sequence of ECG deflections occurring at regular intervals is the hallmark of sinus rhythm.

Standard times

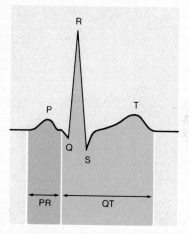

P wave	0.06–0.10 seconds
PR interval	0.12–0.20 seconds
QRS complex	0.08–0.10 seconds
QT interval	0.35–0.42 seconds

Fig.3 Note that the PR and QT intervals are both rate dependent and tend to shorten as the heart rate increases.

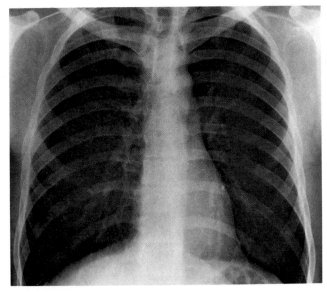

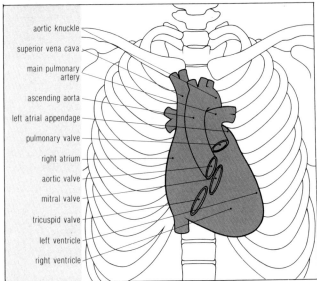

aortic knuckle

superior vena cava

main pulmonary artery

ascending aorta

left atrial appendage

pulmonary valve

right atrium

aortic valve

mitral valve

tricuspid valve

left ventricle

right ventricle

Fig.4 Chest X-ray. This is the postero-anterior projection. Note that the maximum transverse diameter of the heart should not exceed 50% the transverse diameter of the chest.

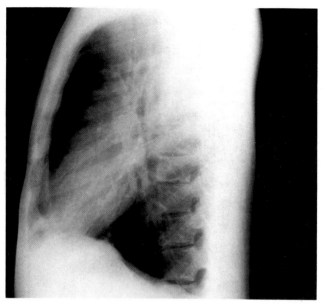

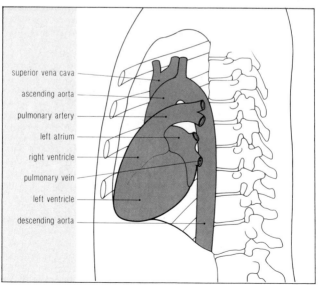

superior vena cava
ascending aorta
pulmonary artery
left atrium
right ventricle
pulmonary vein
left ventricle
descending aorta

Fig.5 Chest X-ray. This is the left lateral projection. Note that the right-sided cardiac chambers lie *anterior* to the left-sided chambers.

4

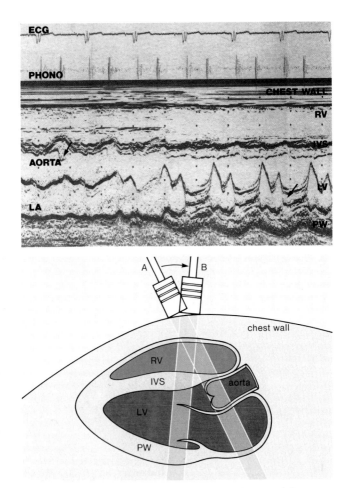

Fig.6 M-mode echocardiogram. Sweep from aortic root to left ventricular cavity. The ultrasound beam provides a one-dimensional 'ice-pick' image of the heart in systole and diastole. The vertical dots are a 1cm scale. Angulation of the beam during continous recording permits sequential examination of the left-sided chambers and heart valves, as shown here. Simultaneous recordings of the ECG and phonocardiogram are shown. The first heart sound correponds to mitral valve closure and the second heart sound (1st component) to aortic valve closure (both arrowed).

RV - right ventricle.
LV - left ventricle.
IVS - interventricular septum.

LA - left atrium.
PW - posterior left ventricular wall.
➝ - points of valve closure.

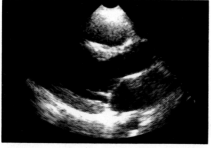

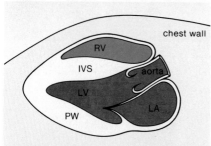

Fig.7 2-dimensional echocardiogram. These are long-axis views in systole (upper) and diastole (lower). The images may be recorded on magnetic tape to provide a 'real time' record of events during the cardiac cycle.
LA - left atrium
RV - right ventricle
LV - left ventricle
IVS - interventricular septum
PW - posterior wall

chest wall

RV

IVS

aorta

LV

LA

PW

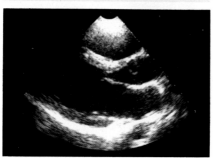

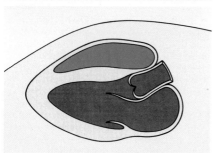

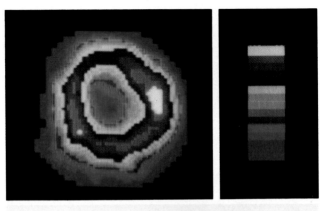

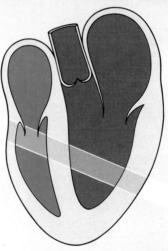

Fig.8 Myocardial perfusion scintiscan. The radionuclide thallium-201 is a potassium analogue that binds to normal cardiac myocytes. The distribution of thallium-201 in the myocardium is closely related to regional coronary perfusion. This illustration is a tomographic 'slice' through the left ventricle, imaged with a gamma camera. Colour coding shows homogeneous distribution of isotope in the myocardium (reflecting normal coronary perfusion) with negligible uptake in the LV cavity. Multiple tomographic slices at different levels may be taken to provide a record of regional perfusion throughout the myocardium. Non-homogeneous distribution of isotope is usually caused by coronary artery disease. Note that isotope uptake in the thin-walled right ventricle is normally insufficient for imaging.

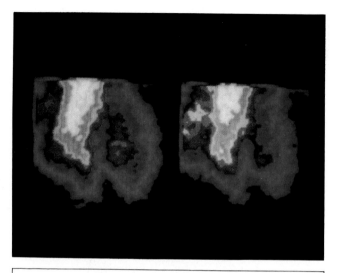

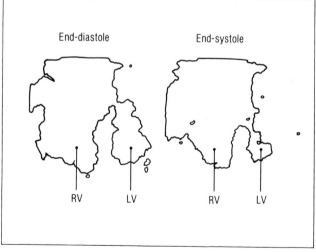

Fig.9 Equilibrium blood pool scintiscan. Left anterior oblique view. Red cells labelled with technetium-99m have been injected into a peripheral vein and allowed to equilibrate throughout the circulating blood. These colour coded images have been obtained with a gamma camera and show the peak and trough of radioactivity within the ventricular cavities after diastolic filling and systolic ejection, respectively. Analysis of wall motion obtained in this way provides a useful index of left and right ventricular function.

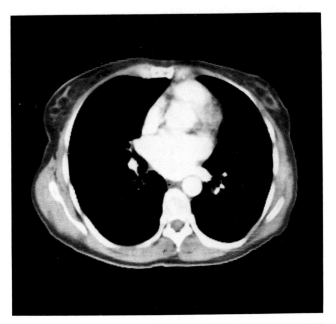

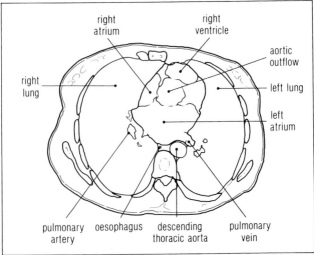

Fig.10 Computed axial tomogram. A thoracic tomogram at left atrial level is shown. The vascular spaces have been 'enhanced' by the injection of contrast solution into the bloodstream.

9

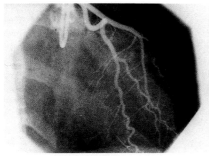

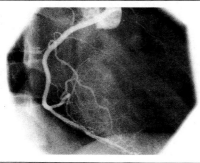

catheter   left main stem

left anterior descending artery

diagonal branch

septal branch

circumflex

marginal branch

Fig.11 Coronary arteriograms. Right anterior oblique views. A catheter has been introduced through the right brachial artery and directed into the ascending aorta. The tip of the catheter has been positioned first in the left and then the right coronary ostium. Contrast material injected through the catheter provides X-ray images of the coronary arterial tree.

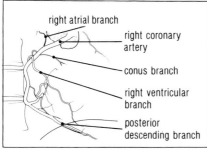

right atrial branch

right coronary artery

conus branch

right ventricular branch

posterior descending branch

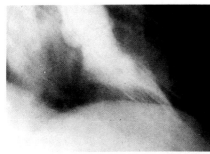

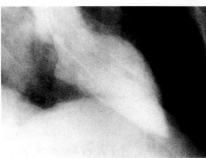

Fig.12 Left ventriculogram. Right anterior oblique views. The catheter has been passed from the ascending aorta through the aortic valve into the LV cavity. These are systolic and diastolic frames from a cineangiogram performed during injection of contrast material.

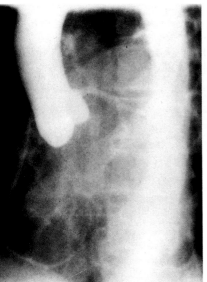

Fig.13 Aortic root angiogram. Left anterior oblique view. The catheter has been pulled back across the aortic valve into the aortic root. A contrast injection provides an X-ray image of the ascending aorta. The coronary arteries arising from the sinuses of Valsalva are clearly seen.

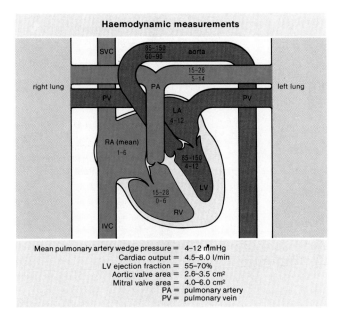

Haemodynamic measurements

Mean pulmonary artery wedge pressure =	4–12 mmHg
Cardiac output =	4.5–8.0 l/min
LV ejection fraction =	55–70%
Aortic valve area =	2.6–3.5 cm²
Mitral valve area =	4.0–6.0 cm²
PA =	pulmonary artery
PV =	pulmonary vein

Fig.14 Haemodynamic measurements. These are normal values measured at rest.

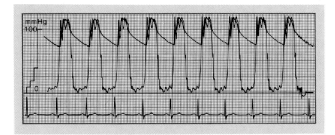

Fig.15 Left-sided pressure signals. Simultaneous recordings of the aortic and LV pressure signals are shown. During systole, LV pressure rises rapidly and as it exceeds aortic pressure the aortic valve opens to allow ejection of blood. Thereafter the pressures remain equal until aortic valve closure occurs. Throughout diastole, the decline in aortic pressure is relatively gradual as blood runs off into the peripheral circulation. LV pressure, on the other hand, falls precipitously and as it drops below left atrial pressure the mitral valve opens to allow ventricular filling. This checks the decline in LV pressure which rises slowly until the onset of systole leads to closure of the mitral valve and initiates another cycle.

12

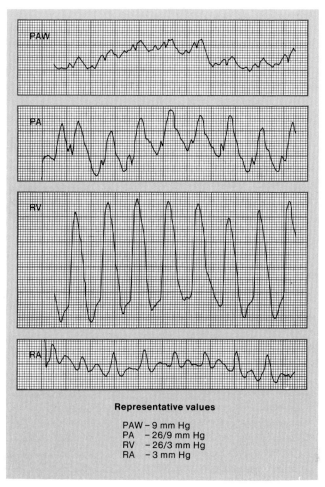

Representative values

PAW – 9 mm Hg
PA   – 26/9 mm Hg
RV   – 26/3 mm Hg
RA   – 3 mm Hg

Fig.16 Right-sided pressure signals. A flexible balloon-tipped catheter (*Swan Ganz catheter*) has been inserted into a central vein and guided through the right side of the heart into a branch of the pulmonary artery. Inflation of the balloon occludes the pulmonary arterial branch and the pressure recorded at the catheter tip (pulmonary artery wedge - PAW-pressure) is a measure of the left atrial pressure transmitted 'backwards' through the pulmonary capillary bed. Deflation of the balloon permits measurement of the pulmonary artery (PA) pressure. Withdrawal of the catheter through the right ventricle (RV) and right atrium (RA) provides a record of the intracardiac pressure signals.

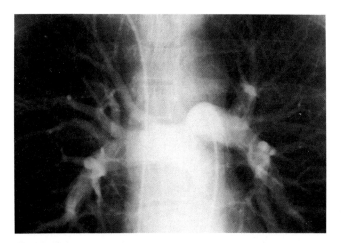

Fig.17 Pulmonary angiogram. A catheter has been guided through the right side of the heart and positioned in the main pulmonary artery. Rapid injection of contrast solution produces opacification of the arterial tree throughout both lung fields.

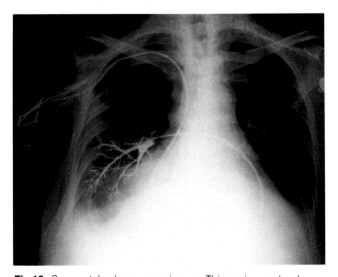

Fig.18 Segmental pulmonary angiogram. This angiogram has been obtained by hand injection of contrast solution through a Swan-Ganz catheter 'wedged' in a branch of the pulmonary artery. The pulmonary vessels subtended by the branch artery are opacified and show a normal fine reticular pattern.

14

ANTERIOR

Perfusion   Ventilation

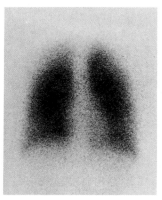 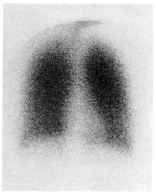

POSTERIOR

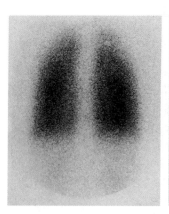 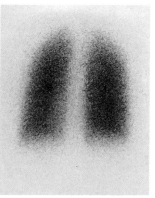

Fig.19 Ventilation perfusion lung scan. In the normal lung, alveolar ventilation and perfusion are closely matched. Inhalation of xenon-133 provides a means of imaging the alveolar ventilation pattern (using a gamma camera) while injection of technetium-99m labelled particles allows the distribution of pulmonary flow to be assessed. This figure shows simultaneous perfusion (on the left) and ventilation scans, viewed both anteriorly and posteriorly.

Coronary Artery Disease

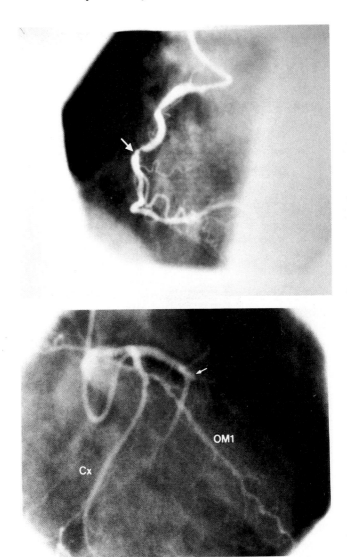

Fig.20 Coronary artery disease - the anatomical substrate. Contrast injections into the right (top) and left coronary arteries are shown. Note the tight stenosis in the right coronary artery (arrowed) and total occlusion of the left anterior descending artery (also arrowed). Irregularities are seen clearly in the first obtuse marginal (OM1) branch of the circumflex (Cx) artery.

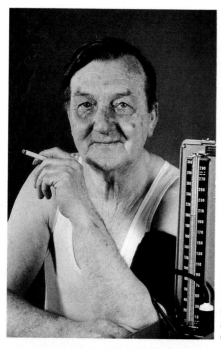

Fig.21 'Risk factors'. Though the cause of coronary artery disease is unknown, a number of factors predispose to its development. Five important risk factors are illustrated by this patient who suffers from severe angina.
1. Male sex.
2. Advanced age.
3. Cigarette smoking.
4. Hyperlipidaemia (note prominent xanthelasmata around the eyes and tendon xanthomas on the knuckles of the left hand).
5. Hypertension.
Other risk factors include a family history of coronary artery disease and diabetes mellitus.

Clinical manifestations of coronary artery disease

Fig.22 Clinical manifestations of coronary artery disease.

1.　Angina

2.　Myocardial infarction

3.　Sudden death

4.　Cardiac arrhythmias

5.　Heart failure

Angina

Myocardial ischaemia results from an imbalance between myocardial oxygen supply and demand and produces chest pain called angina. The pain is usually described as a retrosternal constricting discomfort and occurs in response to stimuli which increase myocardial oxygen demand - in particular physical exertion and heightened emotion. The diseased coronary arteries are unable to meet the extra demand for oxygenated blood and angina is experienced by the patient. The symptoms may be worse in cold weather or after a heavy meal and are relieved by resting. This pattern of symptoms is termed stable angina and must be distinguished from unstable angina in which prolonged episodes of chest pain occur at rest with no obvious precipitating factors. Patients with unstable angina often have critical coronary stenoses and are at high risk of developing myocardial infarction.

Diagnosis of stable angina

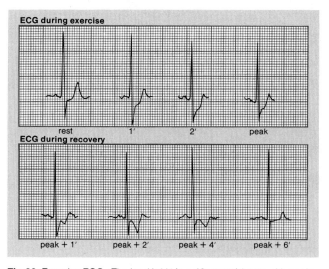

Fig.23 Exercise ECG. The lead is V4 in a 40 year old man with angina who has been exercised on a treadmill. Note the progressive planar depression of the ST segment as peak exercise is approached. During the recovery period inversion of the T wave is seen but after six minutes rest the ECG has almost reverted to normal. In patients with chest pain ST segment depression in excess of 1mm during exercise is highly predictive of underlying coronary artery disease.

18

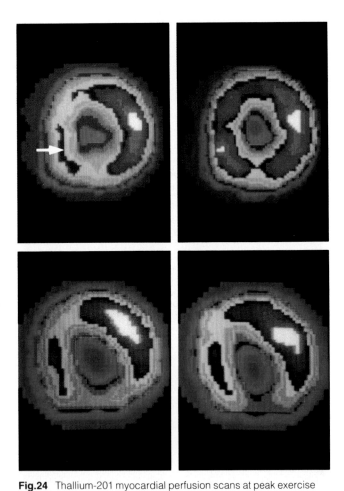

Fig.24 Thallium-201 myocardial perfusion scans at peak exercise and after three hours rest (redistribution scan).
Upper: Reversible myocardial ischaemia. The scan at peak exercise shows a clear defect in the septum (arrowed) indicating impaired perfusion. After three hours rest, however, the defect has disappeared, indicating that the ischaemia is reversible. Thus the coronary supply to this part of the myocardium is restricted but not absent. Ischaemia of this type results in angina.
Lower: Irreversible perfusion defects. The defects in the septum and inferior wall present at peak exercise show no tendency to disappear after three hours rest. This indicates irreversible myocardial damage due to previous infarction. Areas of irreversible damage do not give rise to angina since the tissue is necrosed.

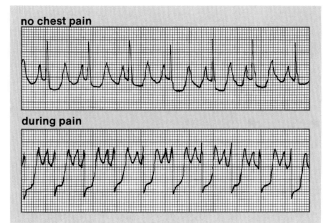

Fig.25 Unstable angina. During chest pain the heart rate increases and marked depression of the ST segment occurs with some loss of R wave amplitude. These changes reverse as chest pain is relieved. Stress testing is contraindicated and unnecessary in patients with unstable angina. The diagnosis is usually clear on clinical grounds and is supported by these typical ECG changes during episodes of chest pain.

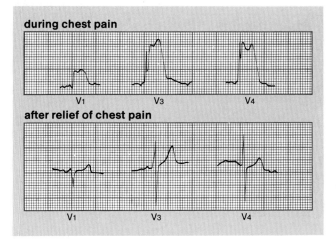

Fig.26 Prinzmetal's angina - ECG. A small group of patients exhibit reversible ST segment *elevation* during chest pain. This type of unstable angina is caused by episodic coronary arterial spasm often without significant underlying coronary artery disease.

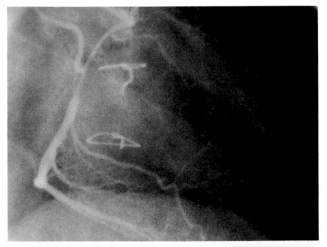

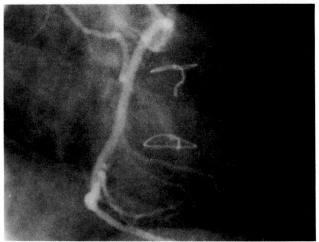

Fig.27 Coronary artery spasm - the anatomical substrate. This patient who had previously undergone mitral valve surgery was complaining of intermittent chest pain occurring at rest. Coronary arteriography demonstrated severe spasm of the right coronary artery.
Top: A long segment of the proximal right coronary artery is severely narrowed.
Bottom: Intracoronary nitroglycerin corrects the abnormality and reveals a normal right coronary artery. The response to nitroglycerin confirms that the narrowing was caused by spasm.

Treatment of coronary artery disease

Medical measures

a. Reversal of established risk factors

b. Drugs: nitrates
beta adrenoreceptor blockers
calcium antagonists

Surgical measures

a. Coronary angioplasty

b. Coronary artery bypass grafting

Fig.28 Treatment of coronary artery disease.

Some preliminary evidence indicates that reversal of established risk factors may slow the progression of coronary artery disease. Patients must be encouraged to stop smoking and steps must be taken to control blood pressure and to lower elevated blood lipids by dietary and pharmacological means. Specific drug therapy is aimed at controlling symptoms by improving the balance between myocardial oxygen supply and demand. Thus nitrates and calcium antagonists improve coronary flow and simultaneously reduce myocardial oxygen demand by lowering blood pressure. Beta adrenoceptor blocking agents reduce myocardial oxygen demand by slowing the heart rate and causing contractility to decrease. These drugs all act by separate pharmacological mechanisms such that their beneficial anti-anginal effects are additive when used in combination. When medical treatment fails to control symptoms, surgical measures may be necessary. The effect of both coronary angioplasty and bypass grafting (Figs.29 and 30) is to improve coronary flow and oxygen delivery to the myocardium supplied by the diseased vessel. This corrects angina but does not necessarily improve life expectancy.

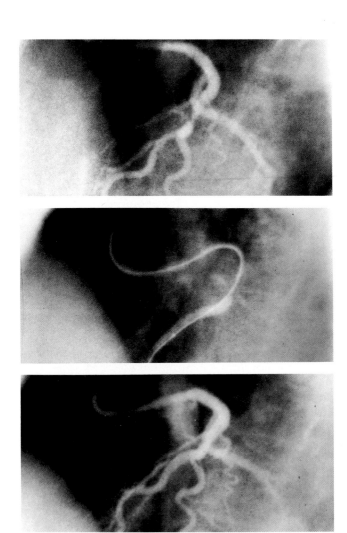

Fig.29 Coronary angioplasty.
a. Before angioplasty. A tight stenosis in the left anterior descending coronary artery is clearly demonstrated. The left coronary system is otherwise normal.
b. During angioplasty. A guide wire has been passed down the diseased vessel and a balloon catheter positioned across the lesion. The balloon is shown here inflated in order to dilate the stenosis.
c. After angioplasty. The lesion has been successfully dilated and the left anterior descending coronary artery is now widely patent.

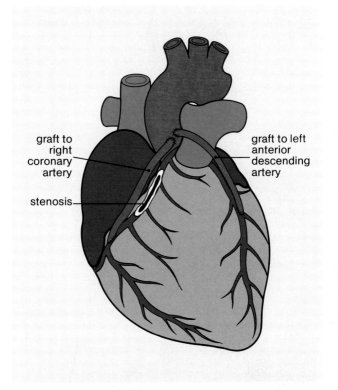

graft to right coronary artery

graft to left anterior descending artery

stenosis

Fig.30 Coronary artery bypass grafting. Segments of saphenous vein excised from the leg of the patient have been sewn into the ascending aorta and used to bypass proximal stenoses in the left anterior descending and right coronary arteries.

Myocardial infarction

When coronary artery disease progresses to complete arterial occlusion the myocardium distal to the occlusion becomes critically ischaemic and infarcts. The extent of infarction relates to the site of the coronary occlusion and the collateral supply to the jeopardised myocardium. Thus a *proximal* coronary occlusion will threaten a greater mass of myocardium than a *distal* occlusion. A well developed collateral blood supply, however, may limit the ultimate damage.

24

Clinical manifestations of myocardial infarction

1. Chest pain – similar in quality to angina but more severe and more prolonged

2. Autonomic disturbance – sweating, vomiting, tachycardia

3. Fever – usually low grade

4. Myocardial damage – praecordial dyskinetic impulse + 4th heart sound

Fig.31 Clinical manifestations of myocardial infarction.

Diagnosis of myocardial infarction
The diagnosis of acute myocardial infarction can usually be made with reasonable confidence on the basis of the presenting symptoms and signs. Confirmation of the diagnosis is made by characteristic ECG and serum enzyme changes. In difficult cases non-invasive imaging techniques can provide useful additional information.

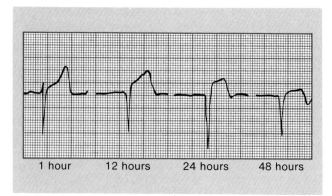

| 1 hour | 12 hours | 24 hours | 48 hours |

Fig.32 Evolution of ECG changes in acute myocardial infarction. The lead is V2 in a 60 year old man. Elevation of the ST segment over the area of the infarct occurs during the first hour of chest pain. A Q wave develops during the subsequent 24 hours and usually persists indefinitely. Within a few days of the attack the ST segment returns to the isoelectric line and T wave inversion may occur.

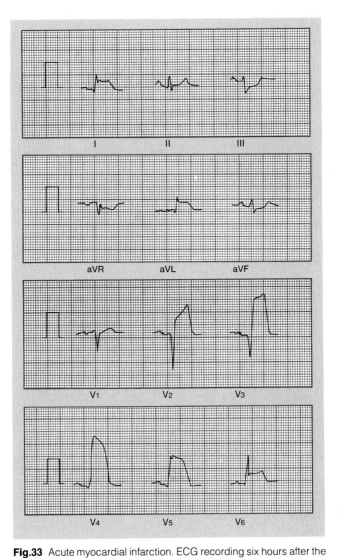

Fig.33 Acute myocardial infarction. ECG recording six hours after the onset of chest pain. Marked ST segment elevation in leads V_2 to V_6 is associated with early development of Q waves in leads V_2 and V_3. Changes in leads I and aVL indicate damage to the lateral wall. Note 'reciprocal' ST segment depression in leads III and aVF. This pattern usually reflects proximal occlusion of the left anterior descending coronary artery.

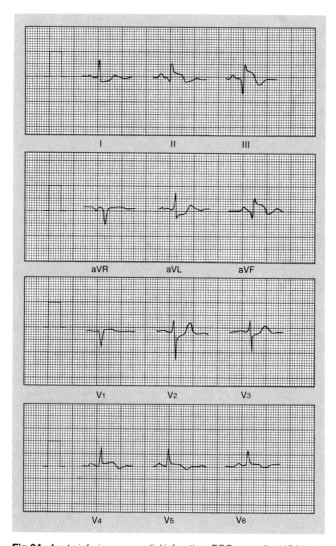

Fig.34 Acute inferior myocardial infarction. ECG recording 18 hours after the onset of chest pain. Typical changes are seen in leads II, III and aVF. ST segment elevation in leads V_4 to V_6 indicates lateral extension of the infarct. Note 'reciprocal' ST segment depression in leads I and aVL. This pattern usually reflects occlusion of the right coronary artery.

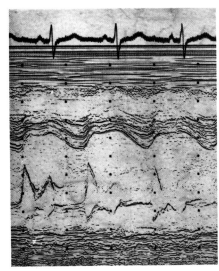

Fig.35 M-mode echocardiogram in acute inferior myocardial infarction (same patient as in Fig.34). This recording shows total akinesis of the posterior wall of the left ventricle. The exaggerated motion of the interventricular septum is a compensatory phenomenon.

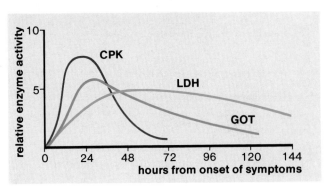

Fig.36 Time activity curves for enzymes released from the infarcted myocardium. Serum enzyme activity is expressed as multiples of the upper reference limit.
1. Creatine phosphokinase (CPK). This is the most useful enzyme clinically. Skeletal muscle is also rich in CPK and false positive results are sometimes found in patients who have received intramuscular injections.
2. Glutamic oxaloacetic transaminase (GOT). The diagnostic value of this enzyme is limited by its lack of specificity. Disease of liver, kidney, brain and lung may all give false positive results.
3. Lactic dehydrogenase (LDH). Peak levels of this enzyme occur late after infarction. Red blood cells also contain LDH and any cause of haemolysis may produce false positive results.

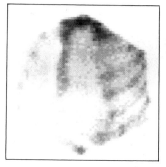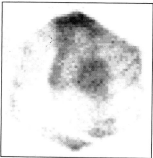

Fig.37 'Hot spot' myocardial imaging. Technetium-99M pyrophosphate is selectively taken up by acutely infarcted myocardium and may be imaged with a gamma camera.
Left: Normal scan. Note that the isotope is taken up by normal bone and the ribs are clearly seen in this example.
Right: Abnormal scan. Isotope has become concentrated in a large anterior myocardial infarct revealed as a dense shadow in the left side of the chest.

Treatment of myocardial infarction

1. Bed rest and ECG monitoring

2. Pain relief – opiates

3. Sedation – opiates, benzodiazepines

4. Anticoagulation – heparin guards against thrombosis in the damaged left ventricle and in the deep veins of the leg

5. Measures to limit infarct size* –
   thrombolytic agents
   vasodilators
   beta adrenoceptor blockers

6. Treatment of complications

   (* of theoretical but unproven value)

Fig.38 Treatment of myocardial infarction.

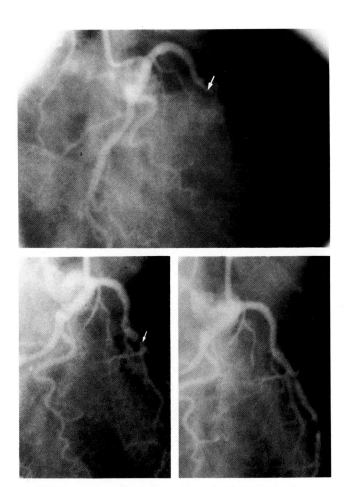

Fig.39 Thrombolytic therapy in acute myocardial infarction. Thrombosis is often the final event leading to coronary occlusion and provides a rationale for treatment of this type. Streptokinase is the most widely used thrombolytic agent.
a.   Before streptokinase. The LAD coronary artery has recently occluded (arrowed), threatening the anterior wall of the left ventricle.
b.   After streptokinase. The drug has been delivered directly into the coronary artery which is now patent but severely stenosed (arrowed). The blood supply to the anterior wall of the left ventricle has thus been restored.
c.   After coronary angioplasty. In order to prevent reocclusion of the LAD, coronary angioplasty has been performed. The tight stenosis has been successfully dilated.

Complications of myocardial infarction

1. Cardiac arrhythmias

2. Heart failure

3. Pericarditis

4. Myocardial rupture

5. Thromboembolism

6. Ventricular aneurysm

Fig.40 Complications of myocardial infarction.

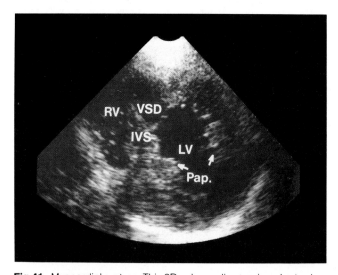

Fig.41 Myocardial rupture. This 2D echocardiogram is a short axis view of the left ventricle (LV) in a patient with anterior infarction. The interventricular septum (IVS) has ruptured to produce a ventricular defect (VSD) communicating with the right ventricle (RV). When rupture involves a papillary muscle (Pap.), severe mitral regurgitation occurs. In either case urgent surgical correction is necessary to prevent death. Rupture of the free wall of the ventricle is nearly always rapidly fatal.

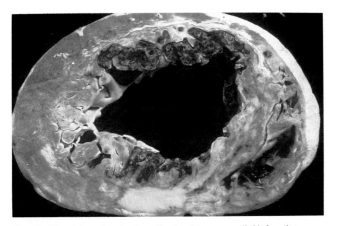

Fig.42 Mural thrombosis. In patients with myocardial infarction, thrombosis overlying the damaged endocardium predisposes to systemic embolism and can result in stroke or organ damage elsewhere in the body. In this example extensive mural thrombosis is seen in a scarred ventricle with recent infarction.

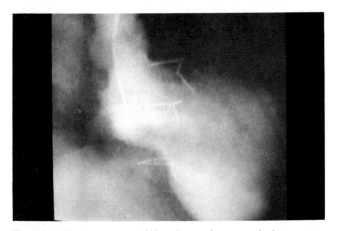

Fig.43 Ventricular aneurysm. LV angiogram in a man who has previously undergone coronary bypass surgery. The aneurysm develops during healing in the postinfarction period. Inadequate shrinkage of the scar results in a fibrotic noncontractile segment which bulges during systole. This impairs the efficiency of the left ventricle and can result in heart failure. Other complications are thrombotic emboli from the aneurysmal sac and ventricular arrhythmias. The development of complications is an indication for surgical excision of the aneurysm.

Adverse prognostic factors in myocardial infarction

1. Advanced age

2. Anterior transmural infarction

3. Left bundle branch block

4. Heart failure

5. Systolic hypotension

6. Complex ventricular arrhythmias occuring late after myocardial infarction

7. History of previous myocardial infarction

Fig.44 Adverse prognostic factors in myocardial infarction.

Apart from the adverse influence of advanced age, the mechanism of which is obscure, the predictors of mortality in myocardial infarction are variably related to extensive myocardial damage and emphasise the important relation between infarct size and prognosis.

Heart Failure

Definition

Heart failure is a syndrome in which a cardiac disorder prohibits the delivery of sufficient output to meet the perfusion requirements of metabolising tissues

Fig.45 This definition is not all-embracing, but it serves to emphasise that the role of the normal heart is to drive the circulation. Any disturbance of cardiac function that undermines this role may result in heart failure.

Causes of heart failure

Ventricular pathophysiology	Clinical examples	Ventricle predominantly affected		
		Left (LVF)	Right (RVF)	Both (CCF)
1. Contractile impairment	Coronary disease	■		
	Cardiomyopathy			■
	Myocarditis			■
2. Pressure loading	Hypertension	■		
	Aortic stenosis	■		
	Coarctation	■		
	Pulmonary vascular disease		■	
	Pulmonary stenosis		■	
3. Volume loading	Aortic regurgitation	■		
	Mitral regurgitation	■		
	ASD/VSD		■	
	Pulmonary regurgitation		■	
	Tricuspid regurgitation		■	
4. Restricted filling	Constrictive pericarditis		■	
	Tamponade		■	
	Amyloidosis			■
5. Arrhythmia	Severe bradycardia			■
	Severe tachycardia			■

Fig.46 Causes of heart failure. Note that the separation of heart failure into LVF and RVF is to some extent artificial, since failure of one ventricle (particularly the left) leads inexorably to failure of both - resulting in congestive cardiac failure (CCF).

Determinants of myocardial performance

Afterload – systolic wall tension

Preload – end-diastolic wall tension

Contractility – inherent force and velocity
of fibre shortening

Fig.47 Preload, afterload and contractility are all terms derived from laboratory studies on isolated muscle. These variables are not amenable to direct measurement in the intact heart. In clinical practice the preload and afterload acting on the left ventricle are usually equated with left ventricular end-diastolic pressure and blood pressure respectively (the variables most amenable to influence by therapy), even though these pressure measurements fail to embrace the contribution that ventricular cavity dimensions make to wall tension. Contractility cannot easily be measured and is usually used qualitatively to describe the inherent force and velocity of ventricular contraction independent of loading conditions.

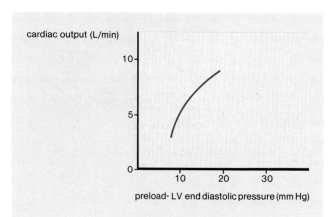

Fig.48 The influence of preload on ventricular function. At around the turn of this century, Frank (1895) and later Starling (1918) described a curvilinear relation between the preload on the heart and the cardiac output. Changes in preload (or ventricular end-diastolic pressure) lead to changes in output in the same direction. The 'Starling curve' has emerged as the major descriptive tool for evaluating the pump function of the heart.

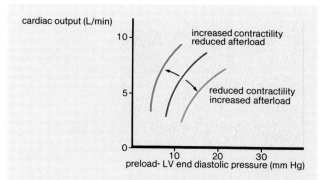

Fig.49 Changes in contractility and afterload influence ventricular function independently of preload. Thus a 'family' of Starling curves may be drawn describing the independent influences of preload, afterload and contractility on ventricular function. At a given preload, changes in contractility result in changes in cardiac output in the same direction, while changes in afterload result in changes in cardiac output in the opposite direction.

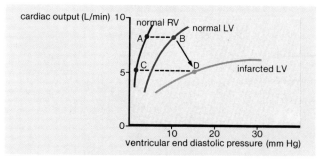

Fig.50 Disordered ventricular function in heart failure. In the normal heart RV diastolic pressure is always lower than LV diastolic pressure, but the output of the two ventricles must be the same. Thus the RV curve lies to the left of the LV curve and the ventricles operate on the same horizontal line (A-B). Myocardial infarction impairs LV contractility and the LV curve shifts down and to the right (see Fig.49). Cardiac output decreases and the ventricles must now operate on the horizontal line C-D. This involves little change in RV diastolic pressure while LV diastolic pressure increases considerably. Thus, in heart failure the discrepancy between diastolic pressures in the RV and LV is variable, depending on the relative degrees to which the function curves are depressed. Measurements of RV diastolic pressure (or central venous pressure), therefore, provide no useful information concerning LV diastolic pressure.

Compensatory physiology in heart failure

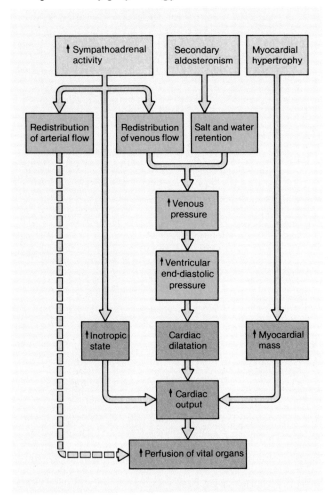

Fig.51 If these physiological responses are inadequate to compensate for the cardiac dysfunction low output states develop, expressed clinically as peripheral hypoperfusion. The situation may be further complicated by the development of systemic and pulmonary oedema in response to critical elevations in venous pressure within the systemic and pulmonary vascular beds. Although the haemodynamic changes that occur in heart failure are complex, *diminished cardiac output and increased venous pressure are the final common pathways for production of virtually all the symptoms and signs of heart failure.*

Symptoms of heart failure

In Figs. 52-54 the points and bars are mean values ±
standard errors in ten patients with LVF. Pulmonary
artery wedge pressure (PAWP) is an indirect measure of
LV diastolic pressure (see Fig. 51).

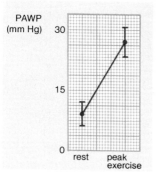

Fig.52 Dyspnoea During exercise PAWP rises steeply. This accounts for the exercise-related pulmonary congestion and shortness of breath that is a common early symptom of heart failure. As heart failure worsens, exercise tolerance deteriorates and in advanced cases the patient is dyspnoeic at rest.

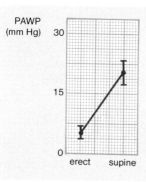

Fig.53 Orthopnoea Gravitational pooling of blood in the upright posture ensures a low PAWP. In the supine posture PAWP rises steeply resulting in pulmonary congestion and shortness of breath (*orthopnoea*), which disturbs normal sleep. In advanced cases frank pulmonary oedema in the supine posture can cause episodes of severe shortness of breath - *paroxysmal nocturnal dyspnoea*.

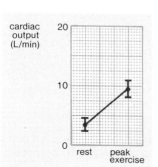

Fig.54 Fatigue During exercise the cardiac output rises to only 9.4 litres/minute - about half the output that is generated by a normal heart. Consequently oxygen delivery to exercising muscle is suboptimal and fatigue develops at an early stage.

Signs of heart failure

1. Low cardiac output	Lassitude Peripheral cyanosis Oliguria
2. Congestive manifestations	Cardiac enlargement 'Functional' mitral/tricuspid regurgitation Basal lung crepitations Pleural effusions Distension of jugular veins Dependent oedema – especially ankles and sacrum Hepatomegaly and jaundice Ascites
3. Sympathoadrenal overactivity	Tachycardia Cool skin Sweating Arrhythmias
4. Other findings	Third heart sound – gallop rhythm Pulsus alternans

Fig.55 In the early stages of heart failure, cardiac output at rest is usually normal due to elevation of LV diastolic pressure and sympathoadrenal activity. Consequently congestive symptoms dominate the clinical findings. Basal lung crepitations, jugular venous distension and ankle oedema are commonly present in association with tachycardia. As heart failure worsens, pulmonary and systemic congestion become more florid and signs of low cardiac output develop.

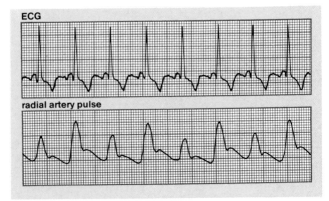

Fig.56 Pulsus alternans. Simultaneous recordings of the ECG and the radial artery pressure in a patient with heart failure. Note the alternating high and low arterial pressure deflections. Pulsus alternans is always indicative of advanced ventricular disease. The precise cause of this phenomenon is not known.

Investigation of heart failure

Chest X-ray This provides a valuable index of the severity of LVF. In mild cases cardiac enlargement (as reflected by a cardiothoracic ratio >50%) is minimal and pulmonary venous dilation - most marked in the upper lobes - is often the only abnormal finding. As failure worsens, cardiac enlargement becomes marked and, with rising pulmonary venous pressure, interstitial and finally alveolar oedema develop.

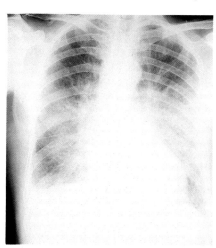

Fig.57 Chest X-ray in acute left ventricular failure following recent myocardial infarction. Note the typical air-space consolidation most prominent in the hilar regions giving a 'bat's-wing' appearance. In this example, bilateral pleural effusions are also present. Because of the acute onset of heart failure cardiac enlargement is not yet marked.

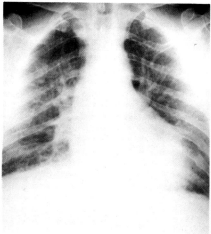

Fig.58 Chest X-ray in chronic left ventricular failure due to cardiomyopathy. The heart is considerably enlarged and the lung fields are congested with prominent upper lobe veins.

Echocardiogram This is the most useful diagnostic investigation in the patient with heart failure. It permits direct measurement of the dimensions of all the cardiac chambers and an assessment of the contractile function of the left and right ventricles. Ventricular wall thickness can also be measured. Equally important the heart valves and the subvalvar apparatus can be imaged. This technique is the most sensitive means available for detecting pericardial effusion. Thus the echocardiogram is potentially diagnostic of many of the common causes of heart failure. Four chamber dilatation and biventricular contractile failure indicates congestive cardiomyopathy. Regional wall motion abnormalities are found in ischaemic disease. Structural and dynamic valvular abnormalities with associated cavity dilatation or hypertrophy (depending on the specific lesion) permits evaluation of the extent and severity of valvular involvement in rheumatic, degenerative, infective and congenital disease. Pericardial effusion is readily detected in the patient with tamponade.

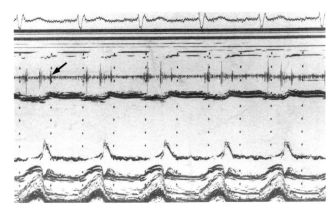

Fig.59 M-mode echocardiogram in heart failure caused by severe coronary artery disease. The heart has become stretched and dilated. Systolic function is severely impaired as reflected by the diminished excursion of the septum and, to a lesser extent, the posterior wall. The phonocardiogram (recorded simultaneously) shows normal first and second heart sounds and also S3 - a third heart sound (arrowed). S3 is a normal finding in adolescence and during pregnancy, but in other contexts it is almost pathognomonic of heart failure.

Radionuclide imaging

This provides an alternative 'noninvasive' means of evaluating ventricular cavity dimensions and contractile function. Technetium-99M labelled red cells introduced into the circulation may be imaged with a gamma camera. The waxing and waning of scintillation counts within the ventricles during diastole and systole permits construction of a dynamic nuclear image (ventriculogram) and enables calculation of ejection fraction. Because isotope decay takes several hours, the technique is of particular value for monitoring serial responses to therapy.

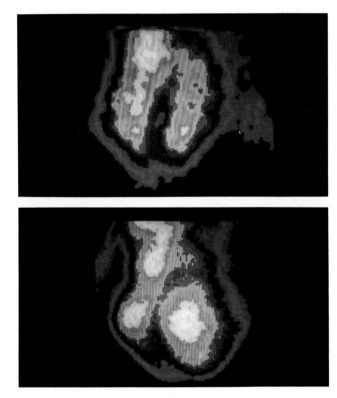

Fig.60 Radionuclide blood pool images in severe congestive heart failure. Systolic (upper) and diastolic (lower) frames are shown. In these 'colour-coded' images the greater the gamma emission the lighter the colour. The dilated ventricular cavities, therefore, most prominent in the dilated cardiomyopathic heart, are represented by the paler areas.

Right heart catheterisation

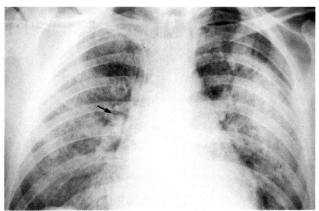

Fig.61 Chest X-ray showing pulmonary oedema. A Swan-Ganz catheter is positioned in a branch of the right pulmonary artery (arrowed). The catheter has a terminal balloon which when inflated occludes the branch to give the pulmonary artery wedge pressure (PAWP), a reliable indirect measure of LV end-diastolic pressure (LVEDP). A thermodilution device permits simultaneous measurement of cardiac output. Pulmonary oedema develops as PAWP rises above 18mmHg and peripheral hypoperfusion occurs when cardiac output falls below 3.5 l/min. Right heart catheterisation is of great value in diagnosing hypovolaemic states causing low cardiac output. In this situation PAWP is low and considerable improvement occurs in response to plasma infusions. The technique also facilitates management of severe LVF and cardiogenic shock.

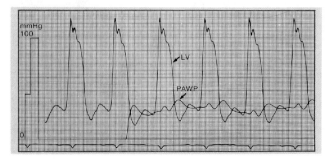

Fig.62 Simultaneous recordings of LV pressure and PAWP. At the end of diastole, just before the rapid increase in left ventricular pressure, LV pressure and PAWP are almost identical. Thus PAWP may be used as a reliable measure of LVEDP. In this example the patient had severe LVF and the PAWP and LVEDP are therefore considerably elevated.

Left Heart Catheterisation

In patients with heart failure, left heart catheterisation rarely provides information that cannot be obtained either by noninvasive techniques or by right heart catheterisation. Its use, therefore, is usually reserved for the relatively small proportion of patients suspected of having surgically correctable lesions e.g. aortic or mitral valve abnormalities, ventricular septal defects, ventricular aneurysms. In such cases the surgeon usually requires precise definition of the lesion and demonstration of the coronary anatomy, particularly in older patients. This information can only be obtained by left heart catheterisation.

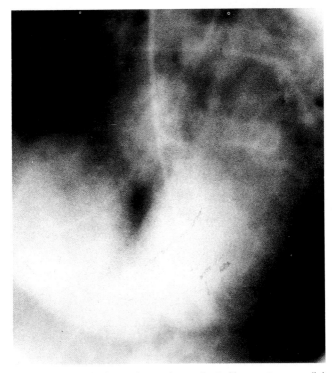

Fig.63 Left ventricular angiogram in a patient with recent myocardial infarction complicated by a ventricular septal defect. Opacification of the right ventricle through the defect is clearly demonstrated. Coronary angiography showed complete obstruction of the right coronary artery. The patient later underwent corrective heart surgery.

Treatment of Heart Failure

Treatment of acute left ventricular failure

1. General measures	Sedate with morphine Nurse in head-up position
2. Correct aggravating factors	Arrythmias, anaemia, hypertension
3. Correct hypoxaemia	Oxygen therapy Mechanical ventilation if necessary
4. Specific therapy	Drugs – diuretics, vasodilators, inotropes Mechanical support – intra-aortic balloon pump Surgery – replacement of diseased valves – closure of septal defects

Fig.64 Treatment of acute LVF.

Drugs used in acute left ventricular failure

Drug	Action	Physiology	Therapeutic effect
Diuretics			
Frusemide (40-80 mg)	Diuresis	↓ Preload	Corrects pulmonary oedema
Vasodilators			
Morphine (5-10 mg)	Venodilation	↓ Preload	Corrects pulmonary oedema
Nitroglycerin (10-150 μg/min)	Venodilation	↓ Preload	Corrects pulmonary oedema
Nitroprusside (25-150 μg/min)	Veno- and arteriolar dilation	↓ Preload and afterload	Corrects pulmonary oedema
			↑ Cardiac output
Inotropes			
Dobutamine (250-750 μg/min)	Sympathomimetic	↑ Contractility	↑ Cardiac output
Dopamine (100-600 μg/min)	Sympathomimetic	↑ Contractility	↑ Cardiac output
		↓ Afterload (low dose)	↑ Blood pressure (high dose)
		↑ Afterload (high dose)	

Fig.65 Patients with acute LVF and pulmonary oedema often respond well to morphine and diuretics. Failure to respond rapidly to simple measures of this type is an indication for pulmonary artery pressure monitoring with a Swan Ganz catheter. Infusions of vasodilators and inotropes may then be given with the aim of adjusting the pulmonary artery wedge pressure to a level that allows pulmonary oedema to clear (15 to 18mmHg) and increasing cardiac output to improve vital organ perfusion.

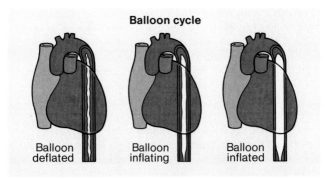

Balloon cycle

Balloon deflated   Balloon inflating   Balloon inflated

Fig.66 Intra-aortic balloon pump. This device may be used to provide temporary support in severe heart failure. A catheter with a terminal sausage-shaped balloon is introduced into the femoral artery and the tip is positioned in the thoracic aorta as shown here. Pumping is sychronised with the ECG such that the balloon is inflated in early diastole and deflated immediately prior to ventricular systole. Coronary perfusion pressure (and hence myocardial oxygen delivery) is thereby increased during diastole and the abrupt fall in pressure that occurs with deflation of the balloon reduces afterload and improves cardiac output. Despite the short-term value of the intra-aortic balloon pump it is often impossible to wean patients off the device. Thus only patients with surgically correctable cardiac lesions are likely to benefit from treatment of this type.

Treatment of chronic congestive cardiac failure (CCF)

1. General measures e.g. salt restricted diet

2. Correct aggravating factors
   e.g. arrhythmias, anaemia, hypertension

3. Specific therapy:

   drugs   – diuretics,
   vasodilators, (inotropes)

   surgery – replacement of diseased valves,
   left ventricular aneurysmectomy
   heart transplantation

Fig.67 Chronic congestive cardiac failure (CCF).

Treatment is aimed at clearing peripheral oedema and improving exercise tolerance. Salt restriction is of some value in limiting salt and water retention in CCF but is usually only necessary in refractory cases. Control of cardiac arrhythmias, anaemia and hypertension is essential in order that maximal pump efficiency can be maintained. Atrial fibrillation is particularly common in patients with CCF and digitalis therapy provides effective control of the ventricular response. Digitalis also exerts an inotropic effect but its therapeutic value in patients in sinus rhythm remains uncertain. Indeed there are no orally active inotropes of proven value for the long-term management of CCF. Thus diuretics and vasodilators remain the drugs of choice. Diuretics reduce the salt and water load and thereby correct systemic and pulmonary congestion. Thiazides are useful in mild failure but the more potent loop diuretics (frusemide, bumetanide) are required in advanced cases. Potassium depletion can be avoided by replacement therapy or by the simultaneous prescription of potassium sparing diuretics (spironolactone, amiloride, triamterene). Vasodilators (prazosin, captopril) also reduce pulmonary congestion by reducing venous pressure. In addition these drugs increase cardiac output by reducing afterload: muscular fatigue during exercise is therefore improved.

Surgery is helpful in patients with valvular disease, left ventricular aneurysms, or septal defects. The majority of patients with CCF, however, have global myocardial disease and heart transplantation is the only surgical option. This is reserved for the most advanced cases who are refractory to all medical therapy.

Valvular Heart Disease

Aortic stenosis (AS)

Causes of aortic stenosis
Calcific disease
Congenital bicuspid valve
Rheumatic disease

Fig.68 Causes of aortic stenosis. With the decline in rheumatic fever in this country, calcific AS - a degenerative process affecting the elderly - has become the commonest cause of AS. Congenital bicuspid valves frequently remain untroublesome until middle-age when calcification usually supervenes.

Clinical presentation of aortic stenosis	
Angina	– ↑O$_2$ demand of hypertrophied LV
Dyspnoea	– ↑diastolic pressure in stiff (*noncompliant*) LV
Syncope	– *either* paroxysmal ventricular arrhythmias *or* exertional cerebral hypoperfusion
LVF	– contractile failure as ventricle dilates
Sudden death	– ventricular arrhythmias

Fig.69 Clinical presentation of aortic stenosis. Note that LVF is a late event which occurs when compensatory LV hypertrophy is no longer sufficient to maintain adequate flow across the stenosed valve. The LV dilates and irreversible impairment of contractile function occurs.

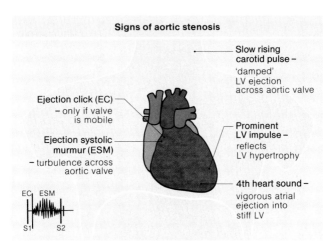

Fig.70 Signs of aortic stenosis.

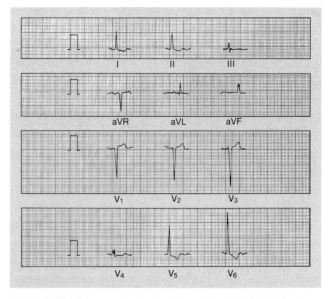

Fig.71 ECG. Note the prominent voltage deflections in the chest leads (V_1 to V_6) associated with T wave inversion laterally (V_5 and V_6). This is a hypertrophy and strain pattern and is typical of conditions in which the LV is subjected to chronic pressure loading e.g. AS, hypertension.

49

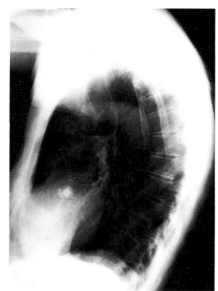

Fig.72 Chest X-ray. Lateral film in severe calcific AS. The calcified valve is clearly visible.

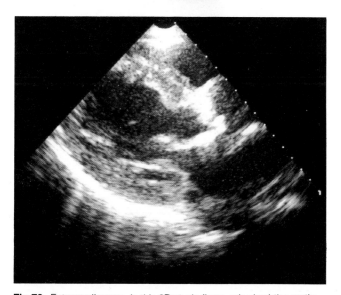

Fig.73 Echocardiogram. In this 2D study (long-axis view) the aortic valve is grossly thickened and highly echogenic. Concentric LV hypertrophy is present.

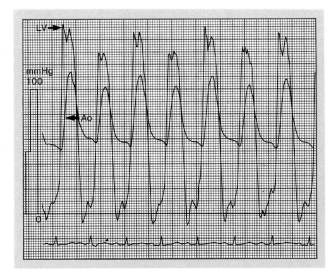

Fig.74 Cardiac catheterisation. Simultaneous recordings of LV and aortic pressure signals. Note that LV pressure is higher than aortic pressure throughout systole. In this example *pulsus alternans* is present - a common finding in AS. The 'size' of the pressure gradient is determined by both the severity of the AS and the flow across the valve. In end stage disease the failing left ventricle is less able to generate pressure: flow across the valve declines and the gradient tends to fall.

Indications for valve replacement

1. Any symptoms of AS

2. ECG evidence of worsening LV hypertrophy and strain

3. Radiographic or echocardiographic evidence of LV dilatation and contractile failure

4. Peak systolic pressure gradient > 50mm Hg

Fig.75 Although AS is well tolerated for prolonged periods, the course is rapidly downhill after the development of symptoms with a three year survival of less than 50%. Irreversible deterioration of LV function is the principle cause of death. Aortic valve replacement corrects symptoms and improves prognosis considerably.

Aortic regurgitation

Causes of aortic regurgitation

Aortic valve leaflet disease – congenital bicuspid valve

– rheumatic disease

– infective endocarditis*

Aortic root dilating disease – ankylosing spondylitis

– Marfan's syndrome

– aortic dissection*

*These disorders produce acute AR. In the remainder
the course is chronic.

Fig.76 Causes of aortic regurgitation.

Clinical presentation of aortic regurgitation

LVF   – contractile failure with severe ventricular

dilatation

Angina – ↓coronary perfusion due to low aortic

diastolic pressure

Note that LVF is a late event in chronic AR

Fig.77 Clinical presentation of aortic regurgitation.

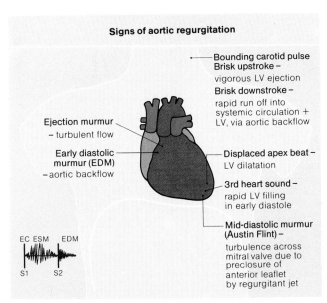

Signs of aortic regurgitation

- **Bounding carotid pulse**
  Brisk upstroke –
  vigorous LV ejection
  Brisk downstroke –
  rapid run off into
  systemic circulation +
  LV, via aortic backflow

Ejection murmur
– turbulent flow

**Early diastolic
murmur (EDM)**
–aortic backflow

- **Displaced apex beat –**
  LV dilatation

- **3rd heart sound –**
  rapid LV filling
  in early diastole

- **Mid-diastolic murmur
  (Austin Flint) –**
  turbulence across
  mitral valve due to
  preclosure of
  anterior leaflet
  by regurgitant jet

EC ESM EDM
S1 S2

Fig.78 Signs of aortic regurgitation.

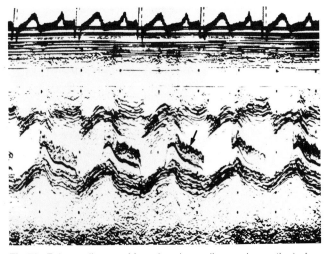

Fig.79 Echocardiogram. M-mode echocardiogram in a patient who presented with acute aortic regurgitation. Dense vegetations (arrowed) are seen on the aortic valve. Gonococcus - a rare cause of endocarditis - was grown from blood cultures.

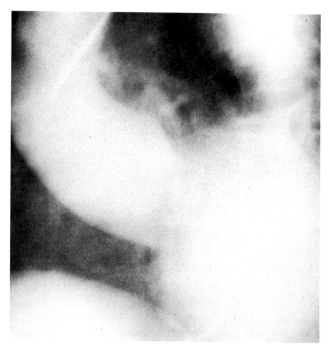

Fig.80 Aortic root angiography. Contrast material has been injected into the ascending aorta through a catheter. Because the aortic valve is incompetent, rapid opacification of the left ventricular cavity has occurred. Note the dilatation of the proximal aorta - a typical finding in aortic valve disease.

Indications for valve replacement

1. Any symptoms of aortic regurgitation

2. Radiographic or echocardiographic evidence of worsening LV dilatation and contractile failure

Fig.81 Although the indications for valve replacement in aortic regurgitation are not clear cut, the procedure must be timed to prevent irreversible deterioration of LV contractile function.

Mitral stenosis (MS)

Causes of mitral stenosis
Rheumatic disease
Congenital mitral stenosis

Fig.82 Causes of mitral stenosis. MS is nearly always a consequence of rheumatic disease.

Clinical presentation of mitral stenosis	
Dyspnoea, orthopnea	– ↑ left atrial pressure
Right ventricular failure	– passive consequences of ↑ left atrial pressure
	– reactive pulmonary vasoconstriction
Palpitations	– atrial fibrillation
Systemic emboli	– atrial dilatation and fibrillation

Fig.83 Clinical presentation of mitral stenosis. Because of the risk of systemic emboli, atrial fibrillation in patients with mitral valve disease is an indication for anticoagulant therapy.

Signs of mitral stenosis

↑ JVP – RV failure

Prominent RV impulse – RV failure

Loud S1 – late closure of MV leaflets at onset of systole

Early diastolic opening snap (OS) – forceful opening of MV due to ↑ LA pressure

Mid diastolic murmur (MDM) with presystolic accentuation in sinus rhythm – turbulent flow across mitral valve accentuated by atrial systole

OS MDM

S1+

Fig.84 Signs of mitral stenosis.

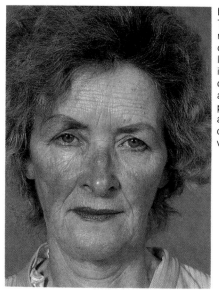

Fig.85 Mitral facies. The pronounced malar discoloration is commonly present in long standing MS but is not specific for this condition. It is usually attributed to peripheral cyanosis associated with low cardiac output and vasoconstriction.

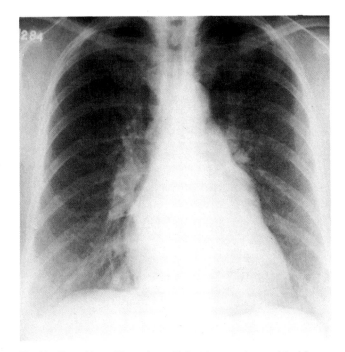

Fig.86 Chest X-ray. The enlarged left atrium produces a 'double contour' to the right heart border and prominence of the left heart border below the main pulmonary artery. Dilatation of the upper lobe pulmonary veins (reflecting elevated left atrial pressure) is clearly visible.

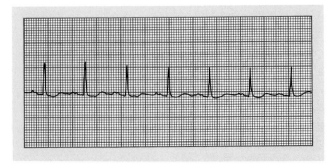

Fig.87 ECG. Lead II showing typical bifid P waves which occur as a result of left atrial dilatation. As the condition progresses atrial fibrillation usually supervenes.

57

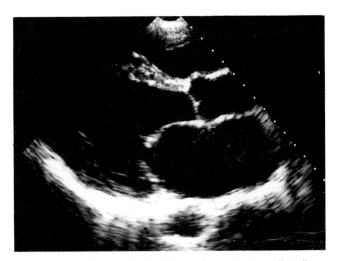

Fig.88 Echocardiogram. In this 2D study (long axis view -diastolic frame) the thickened mitral valve leaflets are poorly separated restricting flow across the valve. Raised pressure within the dilated atrium causes 'doming' of the mitral valve leaflets.

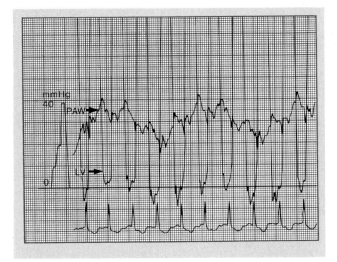

Fig.89 Cardiac catheterisation. Simultaneous recordings of LV and pulmonary artery wedge (=left atrial) pressure signals. Note that left atrial pressure is higher than LV pressure throughout diastole. The rhythm is atrial fibrillation.

Mitral regurgitation (MR)

Causes of mitral regurgitation

Mitral valve leaflet disease	– mitral valve prolapse
	– rheumatic disease
	– endocarditis*
Subvalvar disease	– chordal rupture*
	– papillary muscle dysfunction
	– papillary muscle rupture*
Dilating LV disease	– LVF ('functional' mitral regurgitation)

*These disorders produce acute mitral regurgitation.

Fig.90 Causes of mitral regurgitation.

Clinical presentation of mitral regurgitation

Dyspnoea	– ↑ left atrial pressure, particularly during exertion
LVF	– contractile failure with severe ventricular dilatation
RVF	– passive consequence of ↑ left atrial pressure
Systemic emboli	– atrial dilatation and fibrillation.

Fig.91 Clinical presentation of mitral regurgitation. Note that frank LVF is a late event in chronic mitral regurgitation. Because of the risk of systemic emboli, atrial fibrillation in patients with mitral valve disease is an indication for anticoagulant therapy.

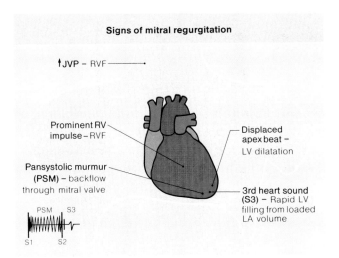

Signs of mitral regurgitation

↑JVP – RVF ────────────→

Prominent RV
impulse – RVF

Pansystolic murmur
(PSM) – backflow
through mitral valve

Displaced
apex beat –
LV dilatation

3rd heart sound
(S3) – Rapid LV
filling from loaded
LA volume

PSM   S3

S1   S2

Fig.92 Signs of mitral regurgitation

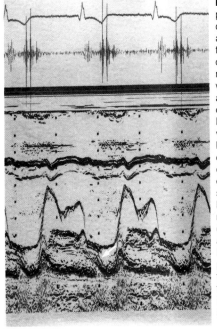

Fig.93 Mitral valve prolapse. This is a common and usually asymptomatic condition. The cause is often unknown but it may be associated with many cardiac and systemic disorders. Systolic prolapse of one or both valve leaflets into the left atrium produces a click and a variable degree of MR. The echocardiogram shows systolic prolapse of the posterior mitral leaflet (arrowed). The click and murmur have been recorded on the phonocardiogram. In this case two additional clicks of greater intensity occur later in systole.

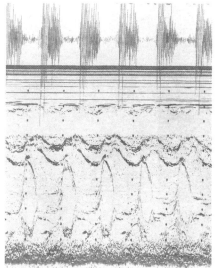

Fig.94 Echocardiogram. M-mode echocardiogram with simultaneous phonocardiogram in a patient with chordal rupture and severe MR. The pansystolic murmur has been recorded on the phonocardiogram. Note the wide excursion of the mitral valve leaflets during diastole, and the vigorous contraction of the somewhat dilated LV.

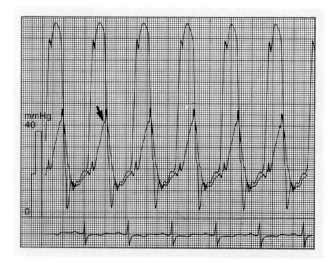

Fig.95 Cardiac catheterisation in severe MR. Simultaneous recordings of LV and PAW (=left atrial) pressure signals. During systole, mitral backflow produces a rapid rise in left atrial pressure as reflected by the giant 'V' wave (arrowed) on the wedge trace.

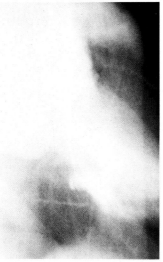

Fig.96 LV angiogram. Contrast material injected into the left ventricle rapidly opacifies the dilated left atrium due to backflow across the diseased mitral valve.

Indications for mitral valve surgery (and surgical procedures)

Symptoms	– effort-related dyspnoea not controlled by therapy
Catheter findings	– significant mitral stenosis (exercise gradient > 12mm Hg)
	– significant mitral regurgitation
Surgical procedure	– commisurotomy for 'pure' mitral stenosis in the absence of calcification and significant subvalvar disease
	– valve replacement for other cases of mitral stenosis and all cases of mitral regurgitation

Fig.97 Indications for mitral valve surgery.

Tricuspid and pulmonary valve disease

Causes of tricuspid and pulmonary valve disease

Pulmonary stenosis	– congenital
	– rheumatic (rare)
Pulmonary regurgitation	– pulmonary hypertension
	– infective endocarditis
Tricuspid stenosis	– rheumatic
Tricuspid regurgitation	– 'functional'
	– infective endocarditis
	– rheumatic

Fig.98 Disease of the pulmonary and tricuspid valve is a rare cause of right ventricular failure. Indeed, tricuspid regurgitation - the commonest right sided valve lesion - is nearly always a secondary consequence of right ventricular failure, which itself is usually caused by left heart failure or pulmonary vascular disease. Primary pulmonary and tricuspid disease can lead to right-sided failure manifested by systemic congestion and low cardiac output.

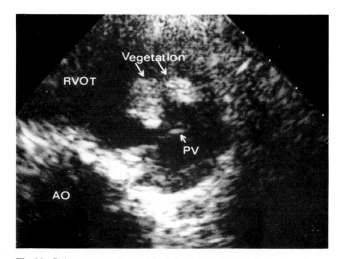

Fig.99 Pulmonary endocarditis. Infective endocarditis of the pulmonary and tricuspid valves is unusual and occurs most commonly in intravenous drug abusers. In this 2D echocardiogram large vegetations are seen on the pulmonary valve (PV). The aorta (AO) and the right ventricular outflow tract (RVOT) are shown.

Myocardial and Pericardial Disease

Cardiomyopathy

The cardiomyopathies are a group of chronic heart muscle disorders which occur in the absence of significant coronary artery disease, hypertension or valvular heart disease.

Congestive cardiomyopathy

Causes of congestive cardiomyopathy

1. Idiopathic

2. Toxic – alcohol, cobalt, doxorubicin

3. Infective – Coxsackie virus, Chagas' disease

4. Endocrine/metabolic – thyroid disease, diabetes, beri-beri

5. Arteritic – polyarteritis nodosa, systemic lupus

6. Infiltrative – sarcoidosis

7. Neuromuscular disease – muscular dystrophy, Friedrich's ataxia

Fig.100 Congestive cardiomyopathy is characterised by global impairment of ventricular systolic function. The heart is dilated with elevated ventricular filling pressures and diminished cardiac output. The majority of cases in this country are idiopathic but chronic alcoholism and infective myocarditis account for a significant proportion of cases.

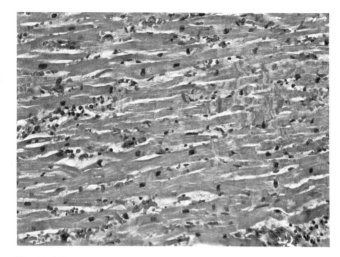

Fig.101 Myocarditis. Ventricular myocardium in acute viral myocarditis showing foci of inflammatory cells and areas with contraction bands. Myocarditis may cause severe heart failure in the acute phase of the illness. More commonly, however, the illness is less severe and is often subclinical. Complete recovery is the rule but a number of patients develop myocardial scarring and progressive heart failure. It has been suggested that 'healed' myocarditis accounts for many cases of 'idiopathic' cardiomyopathy. By courtesy of Dr. C.E. Essed.

Clinical presentation of congestive cardiomyopathy

1. Biventricular failure

2. Systemic and pulmonary embolism

3. Sudden death

Fig.102 Congestive cardiomyopathy usually presents with biventricular failure. Mural thrombi are common within the dilated ventricular chambers and predispose to systemic and pulmonary embolism. These patients are prone to atrial and ventricular arrhythmias and may die suddenly. The ECG and chest X-ray are nearly always abnormal. Physical signs in congestive cardiomyopathy are those of congestive heart failure (see previously).

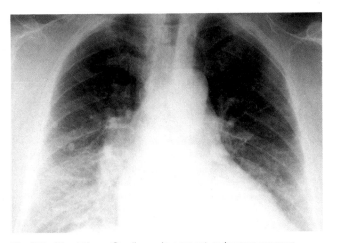

Fig.103 Chest X-ray. Cardiac enlargement, pulmonary venous dilatation and pulmonary congestion are typical features of congestive cardiomyopathy. In this example Kerly B lines are clearly visible in the right lower zone.

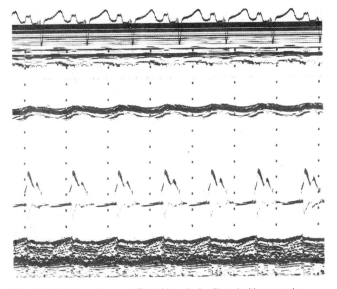

Fig.104 Echocardiogram. The LV cavity is dilated with severely impaired septal and posterior wall contractile function. The patient had idiopathic congestive cardiomyopathy and later underwent successful heart transplantation.

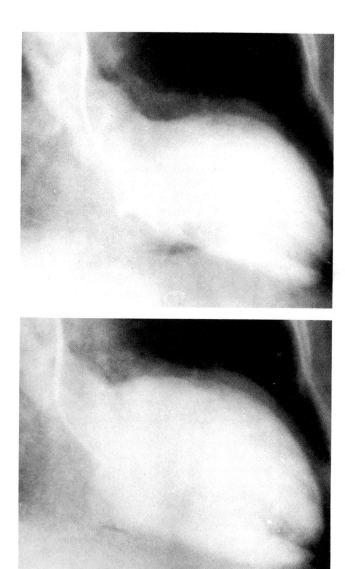

Fig.105 Cardiac catheterisation - LV angiogram. Systolic (upper) and diastolic frames are shown. Note the marked LV dilatation and impairment of contractile function.

Hypertrophic cardiomyopathy

Hypertrophic cardiomyopathy may be defined as primary LV hypertrophy usually with disproportionate involvement of the interventricular septum compared with the free wall of the ventricle. The increased septal mass encroaches on the LV cavity and may cause variable outflow obstruction.

Clinical presentation of hypertrophic cardiomyopathy

1. Angina   – ↑ left ventricular muscle mass

2. Heart failure – impaired ventricular relaxation

3. Sudden death – ventricular arrhythmias

Fig.106 Clinical presentation of hypertrophic cardiomyopathy.

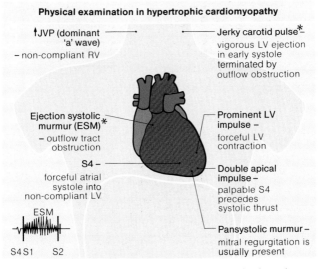

Physical examination in hypertrophic cardiomyopathy

↑JVP (dominant 'a' wave) – non-compliant RV

Jerky carotid pulse* vigorous LV ejection in early systole terminated by outflow obstruction

Ejection systolic murmur (ESM)* – outflow tract obstruction

Prominent LV impulse – forceful LV contraction

S4 – forceful atrial systole into non-compliant LV

Double apical impulse – palpable S4 precedes systolic thrust

Pansystolic murmur – mitral regurgitation is usually present

ESM

S4 S1   S2

Fig.107 Physical examination. Outflow tract obstruction is not invariable in hypertrophic cardiomyopathy and in many cases it is intermittent (see later). Physical signs marked with an asterisk are usually present only in cases with outflow obstruction.

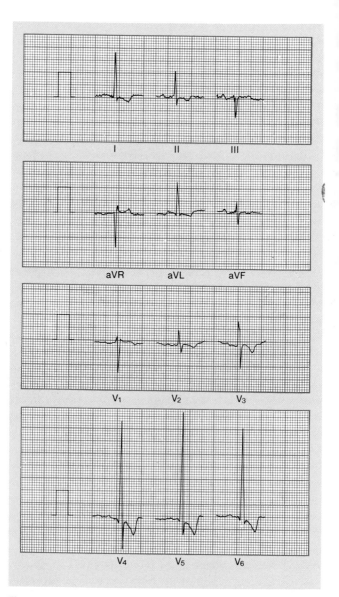

Fig.108 ECG. The ECG is nearly always abnormal in hypertrophic cardiomyopathy with exaggerated voltage deflections and T wave changes reflecting LV hypertrophy.

69

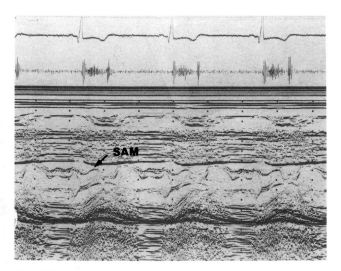

Fig.109 Echocardiogram. Note the massive septal hypertrophy (3mm) with normal posterior wall thickness. Systolic anterior movement (SAM) of the anterior mitral valve leaflet is a typical feature of the condition and contributes to the outflow tract obstruction. The ejection systolic murmur recorded on the phonocardiogram reflects turbulence in the obstructed LV outflow tract.

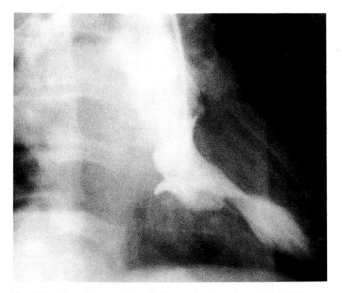

Fig.110 LV angiogram. Systolic frame showing almost total obliteration of the LV cavity in the outflow tract below the aortic valve.

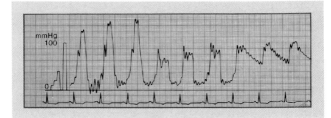

Fig.111 LV outflow gradient. The catheter has been pulled back from the apex of the LV into the aorta during simultaneous pressure recording. There is a systolic pressure gradient (75mmHg) at sub-valvar level in the LV outflow tract but not across the valve itself.

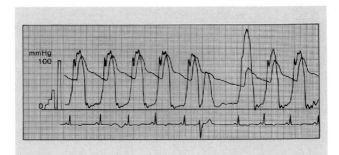

Fig.112 Provocation of LV outflow gradient - ventricular premature beat. The outflow tract obstruction in hypertrophic cardiomyopathy is 'dynamic' unlike the valvular obstruction in aortic stenosis which is 'fixed'. Various manoeuvres will provoke an outflow tract gradient. Here, simultaneous recordings of LV and aortic pressure signals show provocation of a gradient in the beat following a VPB.

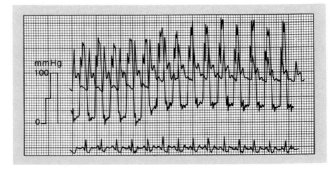

Fig.113 Provocation of LV outflow tract obstruction - Valsalva manoeuvre. Simultaneous recordings of the LV and aortic pressure signals before and during the Valsalva manoeuvre.

Pericardial disease

Acute pericarditis

Causes of acute pericarditis

1. Idiopathic
2. Infective – viral (Coxsackie B, influenza, herpes)
   – bacterial (*Staphylococcus aureus,
   Mycobacterium tuberculosis*)
3. Connective tissue disease – systemic lupus,
   rheumatoid arthritis
4. Uraemia
5. Malignancy – breast, lung, lymphoma, leukaemia
6. Radiation therapy
7. Post myocardial infarction/cardiotomy
   – Dressler's syndrome

Fig.114 Causes of acute pericarditis.

Clinical presentation and physical examination

1. Chest pain – usually retrosternal and 'pleuritic'
   in character

2. Pericardial friction rub – may be audible during any
   part of the cardiac cycle

3. Atrial arrhythmias

4. Symptoms and signs of underlying cause

Fig.115 Any cause of pericarditis may be associated with pericardial effusion. If the effusion is large the heart sounds may be diminished in intensity. A pericardial friction rub does not preclude the presence of a large effusion.

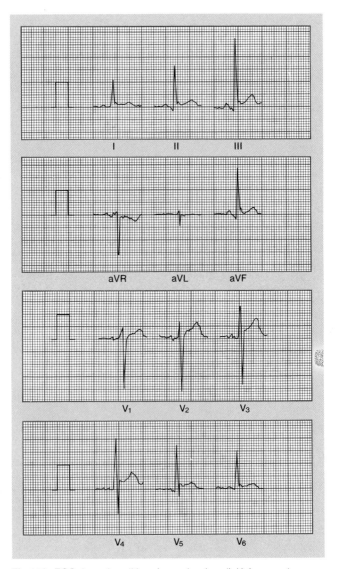

Fig.116 ECG. In pericarditis, minor subepicardial injury produces ST segment elevation affecting any or all of the ECG leads (except aVR) depending on the site of pericardial inflammation. The elevated ST segments are characteristically concave upwards and return towards the baseline as the pericardial inflammation subsides.

73

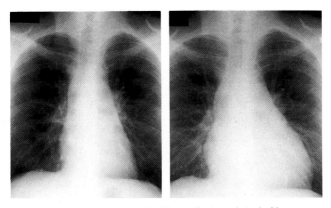

Fig.117 Tuberculous pericarditis. The patient presented with a history of fever and recent retrosternal pleuritic pain. The chest X-ray showed enlarged hilar lymph nodes (left). Cervical lymph node biopsy subsequently confirmed tuberculosis. Two weeks later the heart size was significantly larger due to pericardial effusion.

Cardiac tamponade

Clinical presentation and physical examination

1. Low output state – hypotension, oliguria, cold periphery

2. Tachycardia

3. Pulsus paradoxus

4. ↑ JVP with rapid 'X' descent

5. Kussmaul's sign – paradoxical rise in JVP with deep inspiration

6. 'Distant' heart sounds

Fig.118 Any cause of pericardial effusion can produce tamponade depending on the size of the effusion and the rapidity with which it develops. The gradual accumulation of pericardial fluid permits progressive stretching of the pericardial sac such that substantial effusions may develop without significant increments in intraperi-cardial pressure. Rapid accumulations of fluid, on the other hand, lead to critical elevation of pressure within the pericardial sac. This restricts ventricular filling and causes marked reduction in cardiac output. Urgent pericardiocentesis is mandatory in cardiac tamponade.

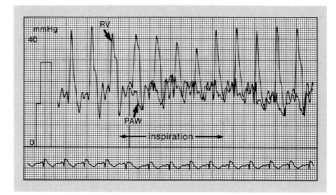

Fig.119 Pathophysiology. In tamponade, intrapericardial pressure rises and restricts cardiac filling. The thin-walled RV is worst affected. A compensatory rise in RV filling pressure occurs which comes to equal LV filling pressure. Thereafter, filling pressures of both ventricles rise together as tamponade increases. This illustration shows simultaneous recordings of the RV and pulmonary artery wedge (PAW) pressures in severe tamponade.

Note: 1. Equalisation and elevation of RV diastolic and PAW pressures (the right and left ventricular filling pressures, respectively).

2. During inspiration RV filling pressure *increases* (Kussmaul's sign) and peak systolic pressure declines (pulsus paradoxus).

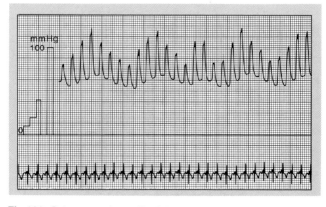

Fig.120 Pulsus paradoxus. Radial artery pressure recording in cardiac tamponade. Note the exaggerated decline in arterial pressure during inspiration. Pulsus paradoxus is nearly always present in tamponade but may also occur in constrictive pericarditis, severe obstructive airways disease and tension pneumothorax.

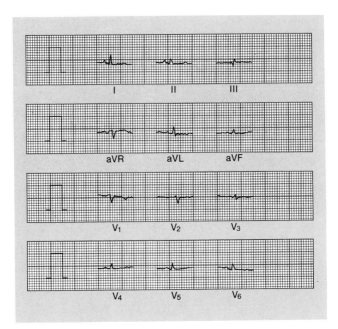

Fig.121 ECG. The voltage deflections in cardiac tamponade are usually of low amplitude due to the insulating effect of the pericardial effusion.

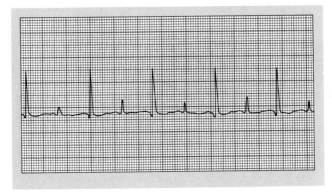

Fig.122 Electrical alternans. This is a relatively unusual ECG manifestation of pericardial effusion and tamponade. The beat to beat variation in R wave magnitude reflects an alternating electrical axis caused by unrestricted movement of the heart within the fluid-filled pericardial sac.

76

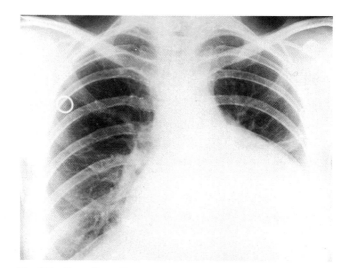

Fig.123 Chest X-ray. The cardiomegaly in this example is the result of a massive pericardial effusion. The following illustration shows the echocardiogram in the same patient.

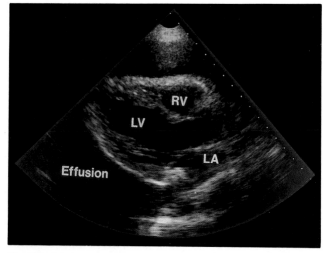

Fig.124 Echocardiogram. This long-axis 2D image confirms massive pericardial effusion. The patient had severe tamponade. Nearly two litres of fluid were aspirated during therapeutic pericardiocentesis.

Constrictive pericarditis

Causes of constrictive pericarditis

1. Idiopathic

2. Intrapericardial haemorrhage – following accidental or surgical trauma

3. Tuberculosis

4. Radiation therapy

5. Uraemia

6. Connective tissue disease

Fig.125 Constrictive pericarditis may follow *any* acute pericardial injury. Tuberculosis is no longer the commonest cause in this country where most cases are either idiopathic or the result of intrapericardial haemorrhage following heart surgery.

Clinical presentation and physical examination

1. Oedema and ascites

2. ↑ JVP with rapid 'Y' descent

3. Kussmaul's sign

4. Pericardial knock on auscultation

5. Pulsus paradoxus (unusual)

Fig.126 Constrictive pericarditis is a chronic wasting illness. Fibrosis and shrinkage of the pericardial sac restricts ventricular filling despite progressive elevation and equilibration of the ventricular filling pressures. Although symptoms and signs of low cardiac output may be present, the consequences of elevated systemic venous pressure and salt and water retention dominate the clinical picture. Treatment is by surgical excision of the pericardium.

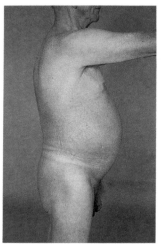

Fig.127 Ascites. This patient presented with severe ascites and ankle oedema due to constrictive pericarditis.

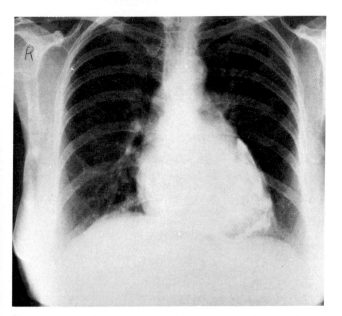

Fig.128 Pericardial calcification. Pericardial calcification may be seen in approximately 50% of cases, particularly those caused by tuberculosis or pericardial haemorrhage. Here it is seen clearly on the postero-anterior chest X-ray but the lateral projection is usually more useful.

Cardiac Arrhythmias

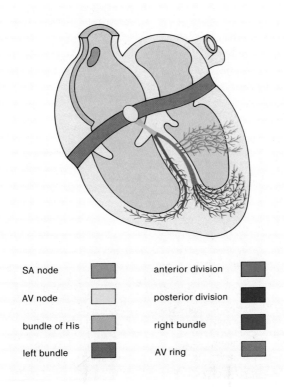

SA node	anterior division
AV node	posterior division
bundle of His	right bundle
left bundle	AV ring

Fig.129 Normal conducting pathways. Synchronised contraction of the four cardiac chambers depends on the highly organised spread of a wave of depolarisation throughout the heart. All cardiac cells exhibit the property of **excitability** whereby a stimulus of sufficient magnitude produces rapid membrane depolarisation followed by a slower repolarisation process. Only the specialised conducting tissues, however, can depolarise spontaneously under normal circumstances. This property which is called **automaticity** is essential to the pacemaker function of the sinus node - the conducting tissue with the highest intrinsic firing rate. The impulse generated by the sinus node spreads first through the atria producing atrial systole and then through the atrioventricular (AV) node to the His-Purkinje system producing ventricular systole. Impulse conduction through the AV node is slow and cannot proceed above a certain rate. This ensures that:

1. There is adequate delay between atrial and ventricular systole for optimal cardiac performance.
2. The ventricles are protected from having to respond to very rapid atrial rhythms.

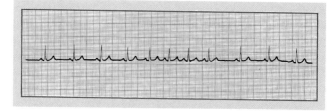

Fig.130 Physiological sinus arrhythmia. Each P wave is followed by a QRS complex and a T wave. This sequence reflects atrial depolarisation, ventricular depolarisation and ventricular repolarisation, respectively. In this example a phasic variation in heart rate can be detected during inspiration and expiration. This phenomenon - common in children and young adults - is termed 'sinus arrhythmia'.

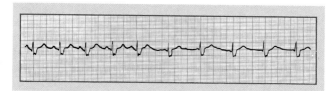

Fig.131 Junctional escape rhythm. The inherent automaticity of the conducting tissue 'below' the sinus node allows it to take over pacemaker function if the sinus node fails. The intrinsic rate of these subsidiary pacemakers is always slower than the normal sinus node. In this example sinus rhythm ceases abruptly after the fifth complex and a junctional (AV nodal/bundle of His) focus takes over. Because ventricular depolarisation proceeds by normal pathways, the QRS complexes of the escape rhythm are identical to the sinus complexes. However, P waves are not seen and the rate is slower.

Mechanisms of Arrhythmias

1. Automatic mechanisms A variety of stimuli - including trauma, ischaemia and drug toxicity - can enhance the automaticity of the conducting tissue below the sinus node and produce isolated premature beats. Automaticity can also be acquired by damaged or diseased cells otherwise not capable of impulse generation. Repeated automatic discharge from an 'ectopic' focus of this type at a rate in excess of the sinus node (or any other established pacemaker) can take over the pacemaker function of the heart and result in atrial or ventricular tachyarrhythmias.

81

2. Reentry mechanisms The basic requirements for reentry are the coexistence of unidirectional block to impulse traffic in part of the conducting system and retrograde conduction via an alternative pathway. This permits the establishment of a reentry circuit in response to premature stimuli. Reentry mechanisms are probably responsible for the majority of sustained atrial and ventricular tachyarrhythmias.

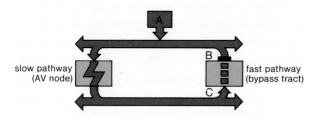

slow pathway (AV node)

fast pathway (bypass tract)

Fig.132 A reentry circuit. This figure illustrates a typical reentry circuit involving the AV node and a fast conducting bypass tract. A premature atrial impulse (A) is blocked at point B in the fast pathway but conducts through the AV node. Thereafter rapid ventricular depolarisation occurs via His-Purkinje pathways and cells immediately distal to the block (point C) are activated. By now the bypass tract is no longer refractory and conducts the impulse retrogradely into the atria thereby completing the reentry circuit and initiating self-sustaining circus movement. The Wolff-Parkinson-White syndrome (Figs.133-135) provides a useful model for reentry arrhythmias.

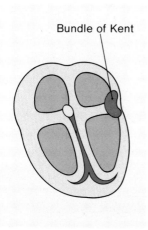

Bundle of Kent

Fig.133 Wolff-Parkinson-White syndrome: the anatomical substrate. Under normal circumstances AV conduction can proceed only via the AV node. The remainder of the AV ring tissue (see Fig.129) will not conduct impulse traffic. In Wolff-Parkinson-White syndrome, however, a congenital anomalous conduction pathway (bundle of Kent) exists between the atria and ventricles. Atrial impulses conduct more rapidly through the bundle of Kent than through the AV node and produce early ventricular activation or *preexcitation*.

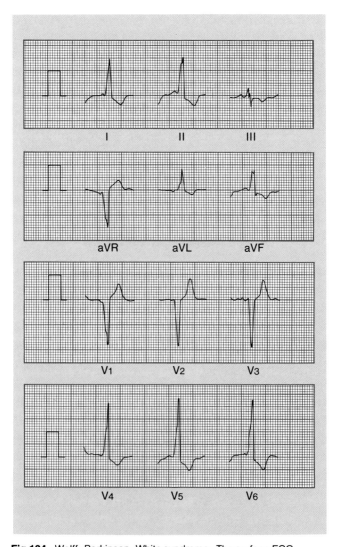

Fig.134 Wolff-Parkinson-White syndrome. The surface ECG. Ventricular preexcitation is reflected on the surface ECG by a short PR interval and a slurred proximal limb of the QRS complex - the delta wave. The remainder of the QRS complex is usually normal because the delayed arrival of the impulse conducted through the AV node rapidly completes ventricular depolarisation through normal His-Purkinje pathways.

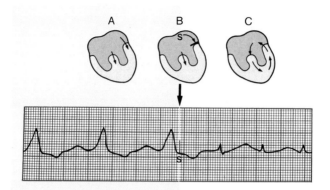

Fig.135 Wolff-Parkinson-White syndrome: reentry tachycardia (recorded at fast paper speed). Just after the 3rd preexcited complex a premature atrial pacing stimulus (S) initiates an impulse that is blocked in the bundle of Kent but is conducted normally through the AV node producing ventricular depolarisation *without* preexcitation. Thus the QRS complex is narrow and lacks a delta wave. The impulse is conducted retrogradely through the bundle of Kent, reenters the proximal conducting system, and completes the reentry circuit, intiating self-sustaining reentry tachycardia (last 3 complexes).

Common causes of cardiac arrhythmias

Cardiac disorders

Coronary artery disease	■	■
Pericardial disease	■	
Mitral stenosis	■	
Aortic stenosis		■
Cardiomyopathy	■	■

Non-cardiac disorders

Thyrotoxicosis	■	
Pulmonary vascular disease	■	
Hypothermia	■	■
Hypokalaemia	■	■
Hypoxia	■	■
Acidosis	■	■

Drug toxicity

Caffeine	■	■
Alcohol	■	
Aminophylline	■	■
Tricyclic antidepressants	■	■
Sympathomimetic amines	■	■
Anaesthetic agents	■	■
Digitalis	■	■
Quinidine		■

Key

Atrial arrhythmias	■
Ventricular arrhythmias	■

Fig.136 Common causes of cardiac arrhythmias.

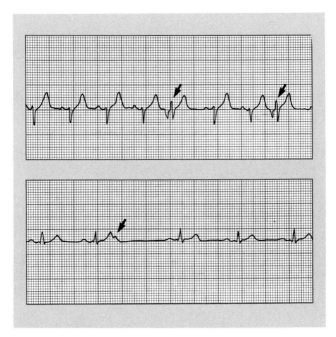

Fig.137 Atrial premature beats (APBs).
A premature and often bizarre P wave is seen on the ECG. The degree of prematurity (coupling interval) is constant in an individual patient for APBs from the same ectopic focus. The premature impulse enters and depolarises the sinus node such that a partially compensatory pause occurs before the next sinus beat during resetting of the pacemaker. APBs are benign and rarely cause symptoms apart from occasional palpitations. Treatment is not necessary.

APBs may exhibit any of the following conduction patterns;
1. Normal conduction - QRS morphology identical to the sinus beats.
2. Aberrant conduction - bizarre QRS morphology (top trace).
3. Conduction with delay - prolonged PR interval.
4. Blocked conduction - advanced prematurity with failure of AV conduction (lower trace).

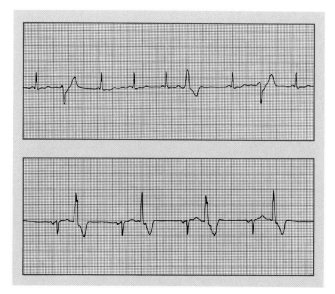

Fig.138 Ventricular premature beats (VPBs).

A premature and bizarre QRS complex is seen on the ECG. The coupling interval is constant in an individual patient for VPBs from the same ectopic focus. The premature impulse may capture the atria by retrograde conduction but penetration of the sinus node is rare. Thus resetting of the sinus node does not usually occur and a fully compensatory pause occurs before the next sinus beat. VPBs are rarely symptomatic but may herald more dangerous ventricular arrhythmias early after myocardial infarction and in conditions such as hypertrophic cardiomyopathy. In these situations treatment is usually given though it is not known whether this improves prognosis.

Upper trace: VPBs from two separate foci. The first and third VPB from a left ventricular focus are morphologically identical and have the same coupling interval. The second VPB from a right ventricular focus has a shorter coupling interval.

Lower trace: Ventricular bigemini. Each sinus beat is followed by a VPB. Note retrograde P waves distorting the early part of the T waves of the VPBs.

Atrial fibrillation (AF)

In AF atrial activity is chaotic and mechanically ineffective. P waves are therefore absent on the ECG and may be replaced by rapid irregular fibrillatory waves. The AV node will conduct the atrial impulses at rates up to 200/min to produce an irregularly irregular ventricular response. Atrial fibrillation requires specific treatment if the ventricular response is rapid because of the risk of heart failure.

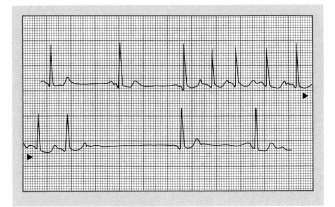

Fig.139 Paroxysmal AF. A six-beat paroxysm of AF follows the third sinus beat. Sinus node recovery is delayed and the penultimate complex is a junctional escape beat before sinus rhythm becomes reestablished.

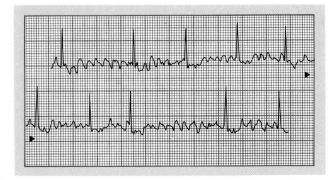

Fig.140 Established AF. Coarse fibrillatory waves are clearly seen with a controlled ventricular response.

Atrial flutter

In this arrhythmia reentry mechanisms produce an atrial rate close to 300 beats/min. The normal AV node conducts with 2:1 block giving a ventricular rate of 150 beats/min. The ECG characteristically shows 'saw-tooth' flutter waves which are most clearly seen when AV block is increased by carotid sinus pressure or by drugs. In difficult cases an intracardiac recording from the right atrium (electrogram) may be necessary to make the diagnosis.

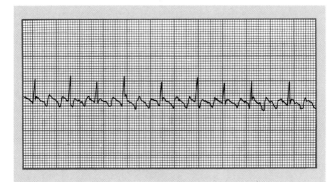

Fig.141 Typical saw-tooth flutter waves are clearly seen. The AV conduction in this example varies between 2:1 and 3:1.

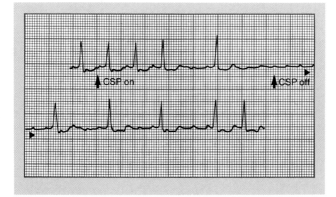

Fig.142 Carotid sinus pressure (CSP) produces vagal stimulation temporarily blocking AV conduction. This reveals unusually low amplitude flutter waves - confirming the diagnosis.

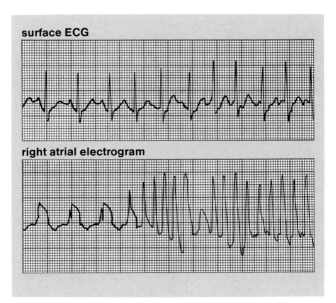

Fig.143 Simultaneous recording of the surface ECG and the right atrial electrogram. After the third sinus beat there starts a rapid arrhythmia. The surface ECG shows a ventricular rate of about 150 beats/min while the recording from within the right atrial cavity shows an irregular atrial rate of up to 400 beats/min. This confirms the diagnosis of atrial fibrillation rather than flutter.

Supraventricular tachycardia (SVT)

This arrhythmia is usually caused by reentry within the AV node with a heart rate of 150 to 220 beats/min. P waves (if visible) can occur before, during or after the QRS complex depending on the activation sequence. If ventricular depolarisation occurs by normal His-Purkinje pathways a narrow QRS complex is produced confirming the supraventricular origin of the arrhythmia. Aberrant conduction or preexisting bundle branch block on the other hand produce bizarre complexes which may be difficult to distinguish from ventricular tachycardia. Treatment is always necessary and is aimed at breaking the reentry circuit so that the sinus node can reassert itself.

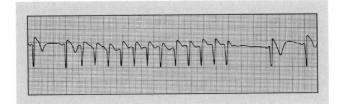

Fig.144 Paroxysmal SVT. After the second sinus beat an APB initiates a self-limiting paroxysm of SVT. Note that the QRS complexes during the arrhythmia are narrow and morphologically identical to the QRS complexes during sinus rhythm. This confirms the supraventricular origin of the arrhythmia.

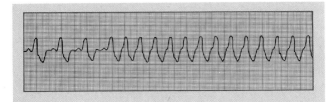

Fig.145 Broad complex SVT. After the fourth sinus beat there is a broad complex tachycardia. Note, however, that the sinus complexes are themselves broad due to bundle branch block and are morphologically identical to the tachycardia complexes. This strongly suggests a supraventricular origin of the arrhythmia.

Accelerated idioventricular rhythm

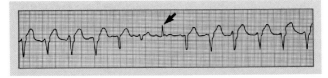

Fig.146 Ventricular rhythms with a rate of 60 to 120 beats/min are included in this category. The arrhythmia rarely occurs except in the context of acute myocardial infarction. The slow ventricular automatic focus is usually in continuous competition with the sinus node such that the idioventricular rhythm is typically episodic and alternates with episodes of sinus rhythm. Specific therapy is not necessary since the ventricular rate is not, by definition, fast and haemodynamic stability is usually well maintained. In this example the idioventricular rhythm is interrupted by 'fusion' beats (part sinus and part idioventricular in origin) and a single sinus beat (arrowed).

Ventricular tachycardia (VT)

VT is defined as three or more consecutive VPBs at a rate above 120 beats/min. Ventricular depolarisation inevitably occurs by very aberrant pathways and the QRS complexes are therefore broad and bizarre. Specific treatment is always indicated not only because of the rapid rate which can produce heart failure but also because of the risk of the arrhythmia degenerating into ventricular fibrillation.

The differential diagnosis from SVT with aberrant conduction can be difficult. The following findings, if present, confirm the diagnosis of VT.

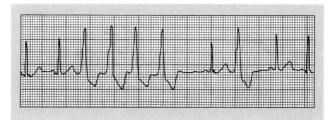

Fig.147 QRS complex during tachycardia morphologically identical to QRS complex of VPB recorded during sinus rhythm. In this example the four-beat run of VT clearly derives from the same focus as the isolated VPB seen later in the recording.

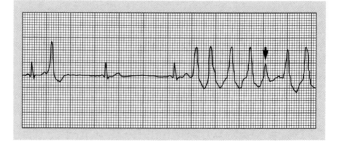

Fig.148 Ventricular capture or fusion beats. During VT, the occasional penetration of the ventricle by sinus impulses will produce either a normal complex (capture) or a hybrid complex representing fusion of the sinus and ventricular beats. Capture and fusion beats must, by definition, occur at a slightly shorter cycle length than the VT. In this example VT is initiated by a very early VPB (morphologically similar to the previous isolated VPB) and is interrupted by a fusion beat (arrowed).

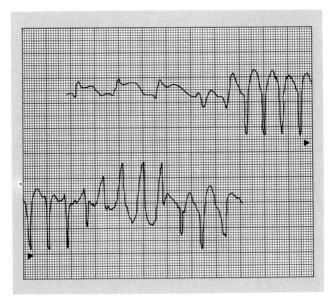

Fig.149 Torsades de pointes. In this example three sinus beats are followed by a broad complex tachycardia. The changing wave fronts (torsades de pointes) during the tachycardia confirm it is ventricular in origin.

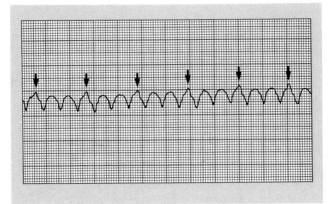

Fig.150 Atrioventricular dissociation. In this example P waves (arrowed) can be seen 'marching through' the VT indicating that the atrial and ventricular rhythms are dissociated and that the broad complexes are ventricular in origin.

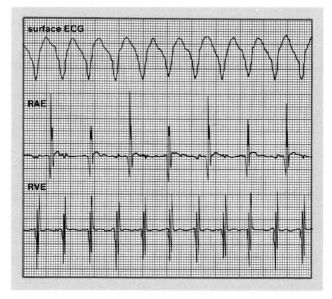

Fig.151 If atrioventricular dissociation is not clear on the suface ECG, simultaneous recordings of the electrograms from within the right atrium (RAE) and right ventricle (RVE) can be helpful. Here the broad complex tachycardia on the surface ECG is simultaneous with the deflections on the RVE, but the deflections on the RAE are slower and bear no fixed relation to the complexes on the surface ECG. This indicates atrioventricular dissociation and confirms the ventricular origin of the tachycardia.

Ventricular fibrillation (VF)

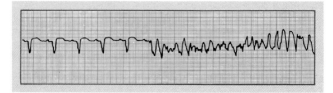

Fig.152 This is a completely disorganised ventricular rhythm characterised by irregular fibrillatory waves with no discernible QRS complexes. VF is incompatible with an effective cardiac output and leads rapidly to death. Urgent treatment is therefore essential. In this example sinus rhythm terminates abruptly with the onset of VF. The patient was undergoing outpatient ambulatory monitoring of the ECG and died suddenly at home.

Treatment of cardiac arrhythmias

Aims of treatment

1. Paroxysmal arrhythmias – suppression of attacks

2. Sustained arrhythmias – *either* conversion to sinus rhythm *or* control of the ventricular rate in cases resistant to conversion

Indications for urgent treatment

1. Critical impairment of left ventricular function

2. Symptoms or ECG signs of myocardial ischaemia

3. Unstable arrhythmias portentous of ventricular fibrillation

Fig.153 Treatment of cardiac arrhythmias

Non-pharmacological therapy

1. Carotid sinus pressure

2. Direct current shock therapy

3. Transvenous pacing – overdrive suppression
   – premature stimuli

4. Transvenous ablation of conducting tissue

5. Surgery – revascularisation of ischaemic myocardium
   – excision of conducting tissue
   – excision of arrhythmogenic foci
   – left ventricular aneurysmectomy

Fig.154 Non-pharmacological therapy. Direct current shock therapy should not be delayed in rapid atrial and ventricular arrhythmias associated with profound reductions in cardiac output.

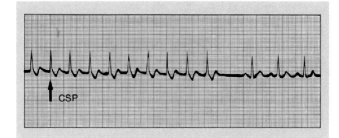

Fig.155 Carotid sinus pressure (CSP). Gentle massage of the carotid sinus produces a reflex increase in vagal discharge. This abruptly slows conduction through the AV node. The manoeuvre is useful for evaluation of the ECG during atrial flutter (see previously). On occasions CSP will break AV nodal reentry circuits and convert SVT to sinus rhythm - as illustrated in this figure.

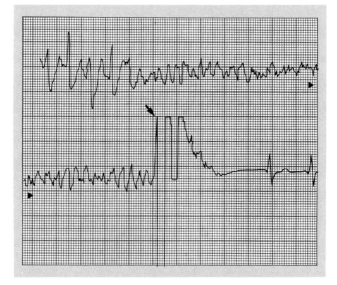

Fig.156 Direct current (DC) shock. DC shock depolarises the entire myocardium and allows the sinus node to reassert itself in the majority of atrial and ventricular arrhythmias. The rapid, almost instantaneous, response to DC shock makes it treatment of choice in those tachyarrhythmias with serious haemodynamic consequences. In this example VT is seen to degenerate into VF. DC shock (arrowed) defibrillates the ventricles and after a short pause a junctional escape beat emerges reestablishing stable rhythm.

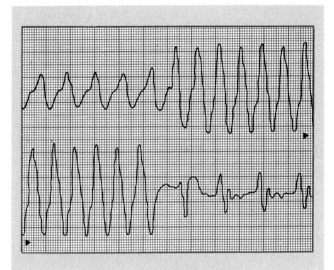

Fig.157 Burst overdrive pacing. This technique can be used for treatment of atrial or ventricular reentry tachycardias. In this example VT (first five complexes) is converted to sinus rhythm (last three complexes) by a burst of right ventricular pacing at a rate in excess of the VT. The pacing impulses penetrate and break the reentry circuit responsible for the VT. This permits reestablishment of sinus rhythm.

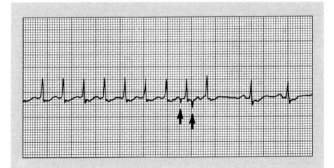

Fig.158 Premature pacing stimuli. This technique can be used for treatment of atrial or ventricular reentry tachycardias. In this example SVT is terminated by two strategically timed atrial premature stimuli (arrowed) which penetrate and break the reentry circuit. Sinus rhythm is thereby restored.

Drug treatment of atrial arrhythmias

1. Blockade of AV nodal conduction	**Control** of ventricular rate in atrial fibrillation and flutter	Digoxin Verapamil Beta blockers
	Termination of AV nodal reentry SVT	Verapamil Beta blockers
2. Suppression of atrial ectopic foci	**Prevention** of all types of atrial tachyarrhythmias	Disopyramide Amiodarone

Fig.159 Drug treatment of atrial arrhythmias. In patients with paroxysmal arrhythmias, combination therapy can be selected with the dual aim of preventing attacks and controlling the ventricular response when this fails. Note that patients with paroxysmal or established atrial arrythmias may be prone to systemic emboli. This is particularly common in atrial fibrillation associated with mitral valve disease when anticoagulation with Warfarin is mandatory.

Drug treatment of ventricular arrhythmias

1. Prevention in acute myocardial infarction	Lignocaine Disopyramide Procainamide
2. Prevention in ambulant patients	Mexiletine Disopyramide Beta blockers Flecainide Amiodarone
3. Termination of established VT	Lignocaine Disopyramide Procainamide Amiodarone

Fig.160 Drug treatment of ventricular arrhythmias. This list is not exhaustive and there are several newer agents not included. Drugs used in ventricular arrhythmias all suppress the automaticity of ectopic foci and the choice of agent is to some extent dictated by its availability for oral administration and its side-effects. Lignocaine, for example, can only be used parenterally and is of no value in ambulant patients. Disopyramide and β-blockers have important negative inotropic properties and should be avoided in heart failure. Procainamide and in some patients amiodarone exhibit long-term toxicity requiring special caution during out-patient therapy.

Cardiac arrest

Causes

    Rapid ventricular tachycardia

    Ventricular flutter

    Ventricular fibrillation

    Asystole

Clinical diagnosis

    Absent arterial pulse

    Unconsciousness

    Apnoea

Management

    Clear airway

    Ventilate – mouth to mouth techniques
              face mask or ET tube

    Initiate external cardiac massage

    Correct acidosis – HCO_3^- infusion

    Correct arrhythmia – VT/VF: DC shock,
                        lignocaine

                    Asystole: calcium gluconate
                    adrenaline

Fig.161 Cardiac arrest. Note that all drugs during cardiac arrest must be given either into a central vein or directly into a cardiac chamber.

Conducting Tissue Disease and Pacemakers

Classification of conducting tissue disease

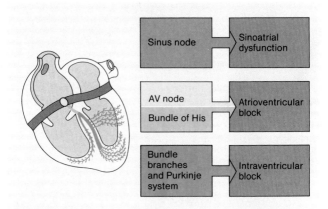

Fig.162 Classification of conducting tissue disease. This classification provides a convenient basis for the clinical and electrocardiographic analysis of conduction defects. It must be recognised, however, that many disorders affect the conducting system at multiple levels.

Causes of sinoatrial dysfunction	
Acute:	myocardial infarction
	drugs e.g. beta blockers and digitalis
	hypothermia
	surgery involving the atria
Chronic:	idiopathic degenerative/fibrotic disease
	congenital heart disease
	ischaemic heart disease
	amyloid

Fig.163 Idiopathic degenerative/fibrotic disease commonly occurs in elderly patients and accounts for the majority of cases of sinoatrial dysfunction seen in clinical practice.

ECG manifestations of sinoatrial dysfunction

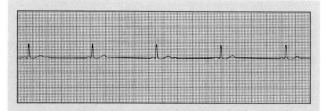

Fig.164 Sinus bradycardia. Sinus bradycardia (< 50 beats/min) is physiological in athletes and in healthy young people during sleep. In other circumstances sinus bradycardia often reflects sinus node dysfunction, particularly when the heart rate fails to increase normally with exercise.

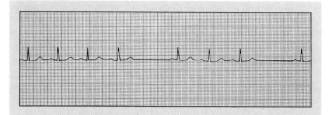

Fig.165 Sinoatrial block. In this example intermittent sinoatrial block (after the 4th and 7th complex) has prevented the sinus impulse from depolarising the atrium. Thus no P wave is seen but because sinus discharge continues uninterrupted, the pauses are each a precise multiple of the preceding P-P intervals. Sinoatrial block that cannot be abolished by vagal inhibition with atropine is often pathological, particularly with pauses longer than two seconds.

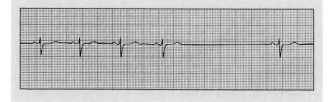

Fig.166 Sinus arrest. Failure of sinus node depolarisation (sinus arrest) after the 4th complex has resulted in a pause which bears no relation to the preceding P-P intervals. Pauses in excess of two seconds are usually pathological, particularly when they occur in the elderly. Prolonged pauses are often terminated by an escape beat from a 'junctional' (low nodal or high His bundle) focus.

Secondary consequences of sinoatrial dysfunction

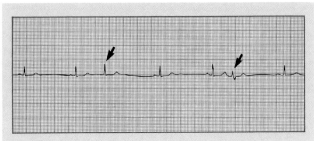

Fig.167 Ectopic beats. Slow heart rates predispose to ectopic pacemaker activity and atrial and ventricular extrasystoles (arrowed) are common.

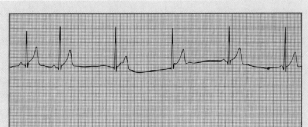

Fig.168 Junctional escape rhythm. After the second complex, abrupt slowing of the sinus rate below the inherent rate of the junctional conducting tissue has resulted in two junctional escape beats, after which sinus node recovery occurs.

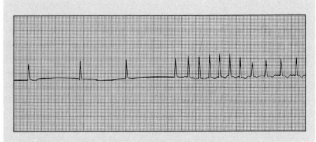

Fig.169 Bradycardia-tachycardia syndrome. In this syndrome chronic atrial (or junctional) bradycardias are interspersed with paroxysmal tachycardias. This example shows a slow junctional rhythm with the abrupt onset of rapid atrial fibrillation.

Clinical features of sinoatrial dysfunction

1. Dizzy attacks and black-outs – caused by extreme bradycardia or prolonged sinus pauses

2. Exertional fatigue and dyspnoea – caused by failure of physiological increases in heart rate

3. Palpitations – caused by extrasystoles and paroxysmal tachycardias

Fig.170 Clinical features of sinoatrial dysfunction

Treatment of sinoatrial dysfunction

1. Pacemakers

2. Antiarrhythmic drugs

3. Anticoagulants

Fig.171 Prognosis in patients with sinoatrial dysfunction is good (particularly in patients with idiopathic degenerative disease) and is not influenced by pacemaker therapy. Pacemaker therapy, therefore, is indicated only in symptomatic individuals to prevent dizzy attacks and blackouts and to improve exercise tolerance. Troublesome tachycardias in the bradycardia-tachycardia syndrome require antiarrhythmic drug therapy. Drugs of this type often exacerbate sinus node dysfunction and a pacemaker may be necessary to protect against severe bradycardia. Systemic emboli from the left atrium occasionally occur in the bradycardia-tachycardia syndrome and some authorities recommend prophylactic anticoagulation.

Causes of atrioventricular block	
Acute:	myocardial infarction
	drugs e.g. digitalis, verapamil
	surgery involving the high interventricular septum
Chronic:	idiopathic bilateral bundle branch fibrosis
	ischaemic heart disease
	calcific aortic and mitral valve disease
	Chagas' disease
	congenital heart disease
	connective tissue disease
	e.g. ankylosing spondylitis
	rheumatoid disease

Fig.172 Myocardial infarction is the commonest cause of acute AV block. Chronic AV block in this country is usually due to idiopathic disease of the bundle branches (particularly in the elderly) though ischaemic heart disease is a relatively more common cause in younger patients. Chagas' disease in S. America, however, is the commonest cause of AV block world-wide.

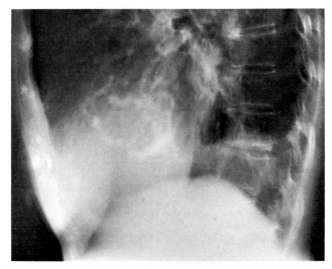

Fig.173 Calcific mitral valve disease. Lateral chest X-ray showing calcification in the mitral valve ring. Complete AV block results from calcific destruction of the lower His bundle. Calcific aortic stenosis may also cause AV block. These are diseases of the elderly.

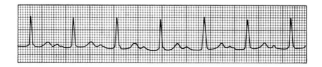

Fig.174 First degree AV block. Delayed AV conduction, as reflected by a prolonged PR interval (> 0.20 secs) characterises block of this type. The AV node is usually the site of block and ventricular depolarisation occurs by normal pathways resulting in a narrow QRS complex. The condition is benign and requires no specific therapy

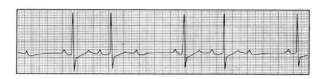

Fig.175 Second degree AV block - Mobitz type 1. Successive sinus impulses find the AV node increasingly refractory until failure of conduction occurs. The delay permits recovery of nodal function and the process may repeat itself. The ECG shows progressive prolongation of the PR interval culminating in a dropped beat. Block is nearly always at nodal level and ventricular depolarisation occurs by normal pathways resulting in a narrow QRS complex. The condition is common in inferior myocardial infarction, is usually transitory and requires no specific therapy.

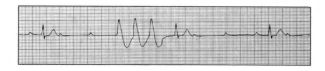

Fig.176 Second degree AV block - Mobitz type 2. Intermittent failure of AV conduction produces dropped beats. The PR interval is constant. The QRS complex may be narrow (as in this example) but is more often broad since block occurs below the junctional tissues in most cases and ventricular depolarisation is by abnormal pathways. Block of this type always indicates advanced conduction tissue disease and may complicate anterior myocardial infarction. There is a significant risk of prolonged asystole. Moreover, ventricular arrhythmias occur in many cases - as illustrated by the short burst of ventricular tachycardia in this example. Pacemaker therapy is mandatory.

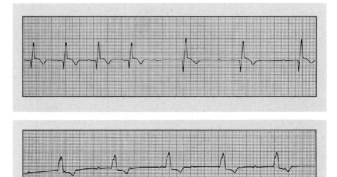

Fig.177 Third degree AV block.

a) Block at nodal level. This occurs in inferior myocardial infarction and also in most cases of congenital AV block. There is complete failure of AV conduction, but a junctional pacemaker with a reliable rate (40-70 beats/min) usually takes over. Ventricular depolarisation is by normal pathways and the QRS complexes are therefore narrow. In this example the ECG (lead III) shows recent inferior myocardial infarction. The first four sinus beats are conducted with a prolonged PR interval (first degree AV block), but thereafter complete AV block develops and a slower junctional focus takes over.

b) Block at His-Purkinje level. This always indicates extensive conducting tissue disease. It may complicate anterior myocardial infarction when prognosis is poor. The ventricular escape rhythm is usually slow and unreliable with a broad QRS complex. Pacemaker therapy is mandatory.

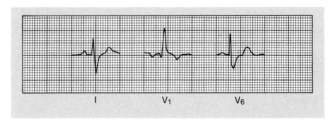

I   V₁   V₆

Fig.178 Right bundle branch block (RBBB). This may be a congenital defect but is more commonly a result of organic conducting tissue disease. Right ventricular depolarisation is delayed resulting in a broad QRS complex with a large R wave in V_1, and prominent S waves in leads I and V_6. No treatment is necessary in isolated RBBB.

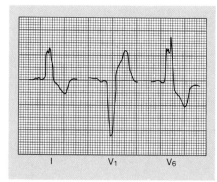

Fig.179 Left branch block (LBBB). This always indicates organic conducting tissue disease. The entire sequence of ventricular depolarisation is abnormal resulting in a broad QRS complex with large slurred or notched R waves in I and V_6. No treatment is necessary in isolated LBBB.

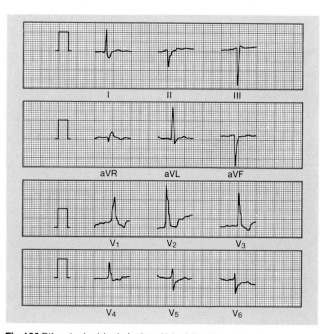

Fig.180 Bifascicular block. Isolated block in either the anterior or posterior divisions of the left bundle (see Fig.129) is called hemiblock and produces left or right axis deviation, respectively. When hemiblock is associated with RBBB, bifascicular block results and AV condition is dependent upon the remaining division of the left bundle. The danger of complete (third degree) AV block developing in this situation is considerable particularly in acute infarction when prophylactic pacemaker therapy is required. In other contexts no treatment is necessary unless progression to complete AV block occurs.

Acute AV block in myocardial infarction

Conduction defect	Incidence (%)	Risk of progression to 3° block (%)	Mortality (%)
None	70	6	15
1° block	5	6	15
2° block			
Mobitz type 1	5	7	15
Mobitz type 2	1	70	50
3° block	7	–	25
LAH	5	3	27
LPH	1	0	42
RBBB	2	43	46
LBBB	5	20	44
Bifascicular block			
RBBB + LAH	5	46	45
RBBB + LPH	1	43	57

LAH – left anterior hemiblock   LPH – left posterior hemiblock

Fig.181   Acute AV block in myocardial infarction.

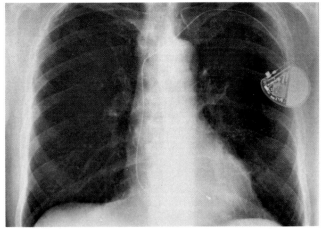

Fig.182 Pacemaker therapy - the equipment
Permanent pacing. The chest radiograph shows a permanent pacemaker system. The power source (or generator) is situated subcutaneously below the left clavicle and attached to a lead with a terminal electrode positioned in the apex of the right ventricle. The generator delivers electric pulses which depolarise the ventricles.
Temporary pacing. Temporary pacing is used when the need for rate control is likely to be only transient (e.g. heart block in inferior infarction) or as a prelude to permanent pacing in patients with severe bradycardias. An external power source is used. This is attached to a transvenous wire positioned in the right ventricle.

107

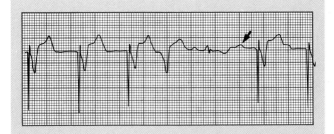

Fig.183 Ventricular-inhibited units are the most widely-used. Here, the first three complexes are paced: the complexes are broad, confirming their ventricular origin and each is preceded by a pacing artefact. A spontaneous ventricular premature beat then inhibits the pacemaker and is followed by a sinus beat conducted with delay (prolonged PR interval). The next sinus impulse (arrowed) is not conducted and the ventricular pacemaker takes over again.

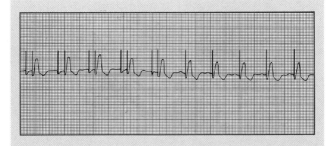

Fig.184 Physiological pacing. Conventional ventricular pacing does not restore synchronous atrial activity in patients with heart block. This is of little consequence when left ventricular function is well preserved but the loss of 'atrial transport' may be important in heart failure. Pacing systems are now available which re-establish the normal atrioventricular relationship by delivering impulses with physiological delay first to the right atrium and then to the ventricle ('sequential' pacing). Alternatively if normal atrial activity is intact 'synchronised' pacing may be used which senses atrial depolarisation and then stimulates the ventricle, again with appropriate delay. Clearly such systems cannot be used in patients with atrial fibrillation. In the illustration the first five complexes are each preceded by two pacing artefacts indicating sequential AV pacing. Thereafter the intrinsic sinus rate accelerates and the preprogrammed pacemaker changes, to synchronised mode, sensing the P wave and delivering an impulse to the ventricle which is thereby depolarised.

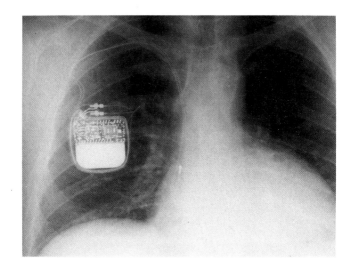

Fig.185 Physiological pacing. Chest radiograph in a patient with third degree AV block and heart failure treated with physiological pacing. The pacemaker generator is situated beneath the right clavicle and attached to two wires - each with terminal electrodes - positioned in the right atrium and the right ventricle, respectively. This system re-establishes synchronous atrial and ventricular activity such that atrial systole occurs at end diastole immediately prior to ventricular systole. This increases ventricular filling and improves cardiac output by Starling's law.

Indications for pacemaker therapy
1. Myocardial infarction (see next table)
2. Symptomatic sinoatrial dysfunction
3. All cases of Mobitz type 2 second degree block
4. All cases of chronic third degree AV block, regardless of symptoms
5. Termination of reentry arrhythmias

Fig.186 Indications for pacemaker therapy

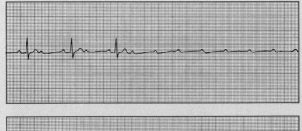

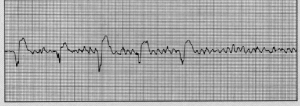

Fig.187 These ECGs provide graphic illustration of the importance of pacemaker therapy in Mobitz type 2 and complete AV block. In the first example, Mobitz type 2 block gives way to complete failure of AV conduction with prolonged asystole. In the second example, the atrium is fibrillating but complete AV block is evident by the *regular* broad complex ventricular rhythm. Again the rhythm strip terminates with prolonged asystole. In both cases a pacemaker would have been life saving.

Indications for pacemaker therapy in myocardial infarction

1. Third degree AV block complicating inferior infarction and any of the following:

   a) Rate< 40 beats/min, unresponsive to atropine
   b) Heart failure
   c) Ventricular arrhythmias requiring antiarrhythmic drug therapy

2. Complete AV block or Mobitz type 2 block complicating anterior infarction

3. Bifascicular block

4. Overdrive suppression of refractory arrhythmias

Fig.188 Indications for pacemaker therapy in myocardial infarction

Miscellaneous Cardiac Disorders

Adult congenital heart disease

Congenital defects commonly seen in adults
Bicuspid aortic valve
Coarctation of the aorta
Pulmonary stenosis
Atrial septal defect (ostium secundum)
Patent ductus arteriosus
Fallot's tetralogy

Fig.189 Congenital defects commonly seen in adults.

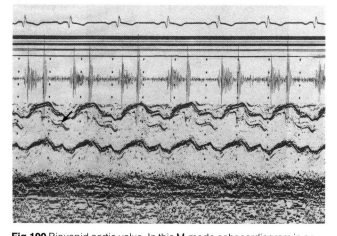

Fig.190 Bicuspid aortic valve. In this M-mode echocardiogram in an asymptomatic young adult the diastolic closure line of the aortic valve (arrowed) lies eccentrically within the aortic root suggesting a bicuspid valve. The valve is normal in other respects. The ejection click and murmur typical of this condition are recorded on the phonocardiogram. Turbulent flow across the bicuspid valve progressively traumatises the leaflets which fibrose and calcify leading to stenosis in middle-age.

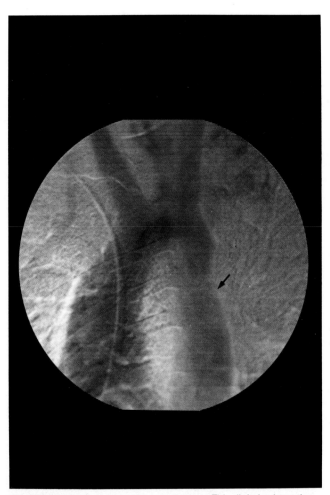

Fig.191 Coarctation of the aorta - aortogram. This digital subtraction study in a young man shows a discrete coarctation (arrowed) in the thoracic aorta. Flow into the abdominal aorta is restricted and the femoral pulse is delayed and diminished. Renal hypoperfusion activates the renin-angiotensin system and leads to hypertension. Death from LVF or cerebral haemorrhage usually occurs in middle-age unless surgical correction is undertaken. Coarctation is often associated with other congenital defects. In this example there was a bicuspid aortic valve (the commonest associated abnormality) which was significantly stenosed. Post-stenotic dilatation of the ascending aorta is clearly seen.

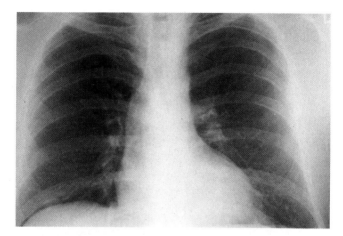

Fig.192 Coarctation of the aorta - chest X-ray. Notching of the inferior aspect of the ribs is the result of erosion by dilated collateral vessels. Other radiographic features (not seen here) may include cardiomegaly and the '3' sign (aortic dilatation on either side of the coarctation produces a 3-shaped contour to the left paramediastinum).

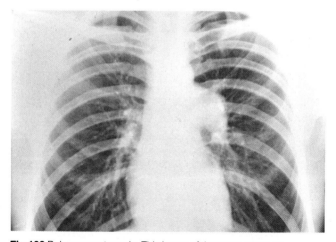

Fig.193 Pulmonary stenosis. This is one of the more common congenital defects occurring in adults. The chest X-ray shows post-stenotic dilatation of the main pulmonary artery and its left branch. Cardiac enlargement and diminished pulmonary vascularity may be present in severe cases. Surgical correction is indicated in symptomatic cases and in cases where the stenosis is very tight.

113

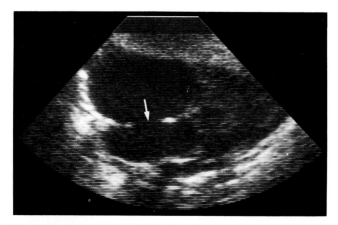

Fig.194 Atrial septal defect (ASD). The 2D echocardiogram is a subcostal view used for examining the interatrial septum. An ASD (secundum type) is arrowed, with free communication between the atria. Blood shunts left to right across the ASD, volume loading the right ventricle and increasing pulmonary flow. Pulmonary hypertension and right ventricular failure supervene in most patients by middle-age.

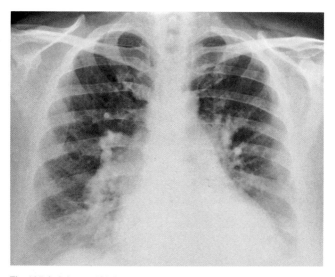

Fig.195 Atrial septal defect - chest X-ray. Note the prominent proximal pulmonary arteries and the pulmonary plethora reflecting increased pulmonary flow.

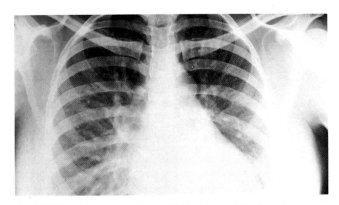

Fig.196 Patent ductus arteriosus (PDA). Failure of the ductus arteriosus closure in the neonate results in a left to right shunt between the aorta and the pulmonary artery. If the shunt is large, heart failure and pulmonary vascular disease develop. Chest X-ray in this adult woman shows a thin line of calcification just below the aortic knuckle. This is the 'comma' sign and represents a calcified PDA. Cardiomegaly and pulmonary plethora indicate that the shunt is large. Surgical correction is necessary regardless of the size of the shunt, because of the risk of endocarditis.

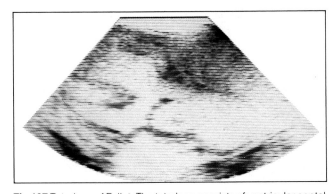

Fig.197 Tetralogy of Fallot. The tetralogy consists of ventricular septal defect, pulmonary stenosis, dilatation and dextraposition of the aorta (which overrides the septal defect) and right ventricular hypertrophy. Pulmonary stenosis is usually severe and increases RV pressure sufficiently to produce right to left shunting across the VSD. This results in cyanosis. In less severe cases the shunt is from left to right (acyanotic Fallot's). The 2D echocardiogram (long-axis view) shows the VSD and the dilated aorta overriding the defect. Complete surgical correction of Fallot's tetralogy is now possible and should be undertaken in all cases.

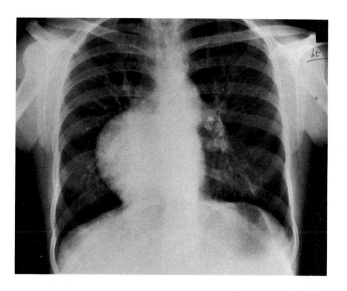

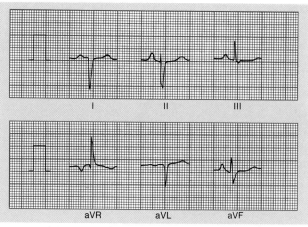

Fig.198 Dextrocardia. The left-sided gastric air bubble indicates that *situs inversus* is not present. Dextrocardia is a rare congenital defect but survival to adulthood often occurs, depending largely on the coexistence of other abnormalities. The chest X-ray and ECG in this example are from a healthy adult. Note that the cardiac apex is situated in the right side of the chest and that the QRS vector is negative in leads I and aVL but positive in aVR. (The positive P waves in I, II and III distinguish this from accidental reversal of the left and right arm leads).

Clinical presentation of aortic dissection

1. Chest pain

2. Regional arterial insufficiency

3. Aortic regurgitation

4. Cardiac tamponade

5. Sudden death

Fig.199 Clinical presentation. In patients with degenerative disease of the aortic media, an intimal tear allows high pressure arterial blood to create a false lumen for a variable distance through the aortic media. The tear is usually proximal, just above the aortic valve, but may be more distal particularly in hypertensive patients. Partial or complete occlusion of branch arteries arising from the aorta leads to regional ischaemia while disruption of the aortic valve ring produces aortic regurgitation. External rupture into the pericardial or pleural spaces is common and often fatal. Where possible, surgical repair should be undertaken, particularly in proximal dissections.

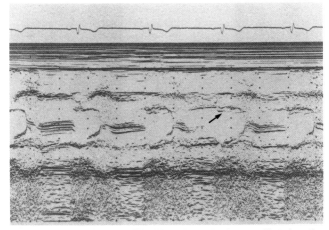

Fig.200 Echocardiogram. This M-mode study shows a dilated aortic root with an intimal flap (arrowed) separating the true and false lumens.

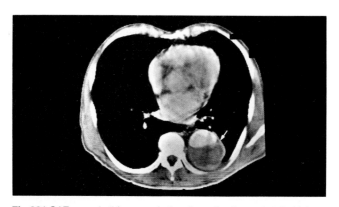

Fig.201 CAT scan. In this example the dissection has extended into the descending thoracic aorta (arrowed) which is considerably dilated. Contrast enhancement clearly separates the true and false lumens.

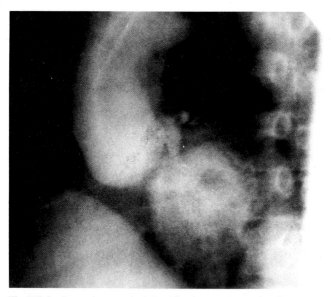

Fig.202 Aortic angiogram. An intimal flap is seen traversing the sinuses of Valsalva (with partial disruption of the left coronary ostium) and passing distally in the thoracic aorta to the left of the catheter Opacification of the LV cavity indicates regurgitation due to disruption of the valve ring.

Pulmonary thromboembolism

Clinical presentation of pulmonary thromboembolism

Symptoms   Chest pain*

Dyspnoea*

Cough*

Haemoptysis

Syncope

Signs   Tachypnoea*

Loud S_2 (pulmonary component)*

Tachycardia

↑JVP

Gallop rhythm

Signs of DVT

Cyanosis

*present in > 50% of patients with pulmonary embolism

Fig.203 Clinical presentation. Pulmonary thromboembolism usually derives from the deep veins of the legs or pelvis. It is a common cause of hospital morbidity and mortality. The severity of the clinical presentation relates to the extent of pulmonary vascular obstruction but the symptoms and signs are very variable and usually nondiagnostic.

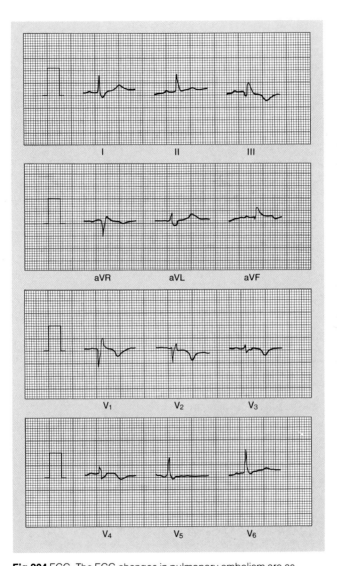

Fig.204 ECG. The ECG changes in pulmonary embolism are as variable as the clinical findings and are nondiagnostic. Classically, however, the changes reflect RV strain as illustrated in this example from a patient with massive pulmonary embolism. Note the S1, Q3, T3 pattern with incomplete RBBB. T wave inversion in V1 to V4 is a further manifestation of RV strain.

ANTERIOR

Perfusion   Ventilation

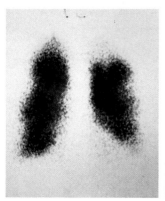 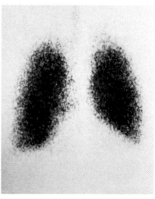

POSTERIOR

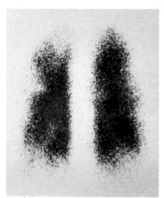 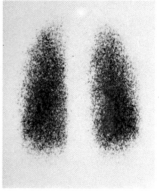

Fig.205 Ventilation-perfusion isotope lung scan. In pulmonary embolism, alveolar ventilation remains normal and the ventilation scan shows homogeneous distribution of isotope. Blood flow to those parts of the lung subtended by the obstructed vessel (or vessels), however, is impaired and the perfusion scan shows regional defects. The demonstration of ventilation-perfusion 'mismatch' is highly specific for pulmonary embolism. In this example ventilation scans are on the right and perfusion scans are on the left. Several areas of mismatch are seen indicating multiple pulmonary emboli.

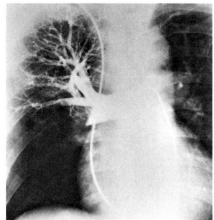

Fig.206 Pulmonary angiogram. There is complete obstruction of the left pulmonary artery and also of the branches to the right middle and lower lobes. Only the right upper lobe branches are patent. The patient had suffered massive pulmonary embolism and later died.

Chronic cor pulmonale

Definition: Right-sided heart failure caused by respiratory disease or pulmonary vascular disease.

Causes of cor pulmonale

1. Obstructive airways disease – bronchitis, emphysema, asthma

2. Parenchymal disease – sarcoidosis, pneumoconiosis, bronchiectasis

3. Neuromuscular and chest wall disease – poliomyelitis, kyphoscoliosis

4. Impaired respiratory drive – Pickwickian syndrome

5. Pulmonary vascular disease – primary pulmonary hypertension, chronic pulmonary emboli

Fig.207 These disorders produce pulmonary hypertension either by destruction of the pulmonary vascular bed or by hypoxic pulmonary vasoconstriction. The right ventricle compensates by progressive hypertrophy but eventually dilates and fails, producing systemic congestion and low cardiac output.

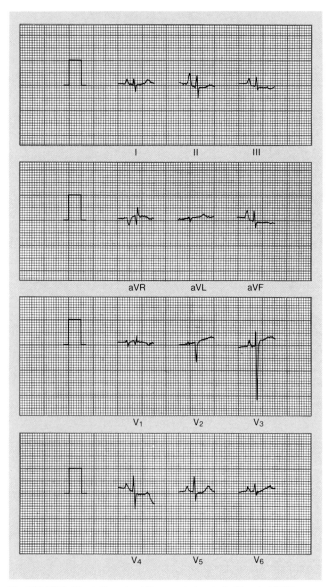

Fig.208 ECG. The tall peaked P waves in leads II, III and aVF (P pulmonale) and the prominent R wave with T wave inversion in lead VI are typical features of right-sided strain in cor pulmonale.

123

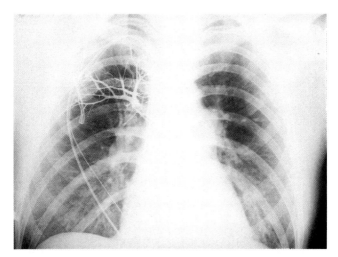

Fig.209 Segmental pulmonary angiogram. Contrast material has been injected through a Swan Ganz catheter wedged in a right upper lobe branch of the pulmonary artery. Note that the normal fine reticular pattern of the pulmonary vessels is lost. The patient had primary pulmonary hypertension.

Classification of primary cardiac tumours	
Benign	Myxoma
	Lipoma
	Rhabdomyoma
	Fibroma
Malignant	Angiosarcoma
	Rhabdomyosarcoma
	Fibrosarcoma

Fig.210 Primary cardiac tumours are rare. The large majority are the histologically benign myxoma.

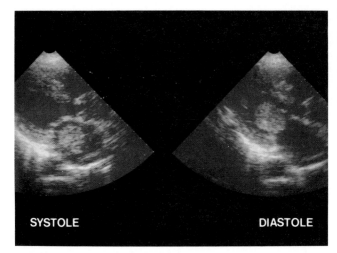

Fig.211 Myxoma - echocardiogram. Although myxomas may occur in any of the cardiac chambers, the majority are left atrial and present with symptoms and signs that are almost indistinguishable from mitral stenosis. These 2D echocardiograms in systole and diastole show a left atrial myxoma. Note that during diastole the tumour prolapses through the mitral valve obstructing LV filling as if the valve were stenosed.

Index

CAPOTEN™

captopril

Prescribing Information CAPOTEN TABLETS ▼ Presentation:
Tablets containing 12.5 mg, 25 mg or 50 mg captopril. **Indication:**
In severe hypertension where standard therapy has failed.
In severe, treatment refractory congestive heart failure. **Dosage
in Hypertension:** Treatment should be at the lowest effective
dose. Initially 25 mg b.d., which may be increased incrementally
at two-week intervals to a maximum of 50 mg t.i.d. If a
satisfactory response has not been achieved, diuretic therapy
should be added. In severe hypertension where patients may be
volume depleted, the addition of Capoten to multiple anti-
hypertensive agents should be initiated under close medical
supervision. **Dosage in C.H.F.:** 25 mg t.i.d. Starting dose of
6.25 mg or 12.5 mg t.i.d. may minimise transient hypotension.
Capoten should be used with a diuretic and where appropriate
digitalis. Patients on high dose diuretic therapy must be started
under medical supervision. **Contra-Indications:** Hypersensitivity
to captopril. **Warnings/Precautions:** There have been reports of
neutropenia/agranulocytosis and proteinuria, but these are rare
in patients with normal renal function. In elderly patients or
those with impaired renal function or with connective tissue
disease, particularly SLE, and in patients concurrently receiving
immuno-suppressant drugs, therapy should be initiated with
caution, and response titrated. Patients should report any
infection and if neutropenia is suspected captopril should be
withdrawn. Neutropenia is normally reversible — see Data Sheet.
Impaired renal function, renal artery stenosis, surgery/
anaesthesia, hypotension, pregnancy and lactation — see Data
Sheet. Hypotension: In patients on high dose diuretic therapy
exaggerated hypotensive responses have occurred usually within
1 hour of the initial captopril dose. Occasional hypotension may
be relieved by the patient lying down. The risk of hypotension is
lessened by commencing therapy on a lower dose. **Side Effects:**
Skin rashes, taste disturbance and gastrointestinal upset have
been reported. These are usually mild and transient. **Drug
Interactions:** See Data Sheet. **Overdosage:** See Data Sheet.
Product Licence Numbers: Capoten Tablets 12.5 mg;
PL0034/0221; Capoten Tablets 25mg; PL0034/0193; Capoten
Tablets 50 mg; PL0034/0194. **Basic NHS price:** 12.5 mg tablets
100 — £16.40; 25 mg tablets 56 — £13.37; 50 mg tablets 56 —
£20.50. **Legal Category:** POM. Capoten is a Squibb Trade Mark.
Special reporting to CSM required. ▼ AO9351. April 85.

SQUIBB™

Further information available on request from:
Technical Services Department, E.R. Squibb & Sons Limited,
Squibb House, 141-149 Staines Road, Hounslow, Middlesex
TW3 3JA. Tel: 01-572 7422.

At the forefront of cardiovascular medicine.